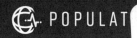

POPULATION HEALTH

A PRIMER

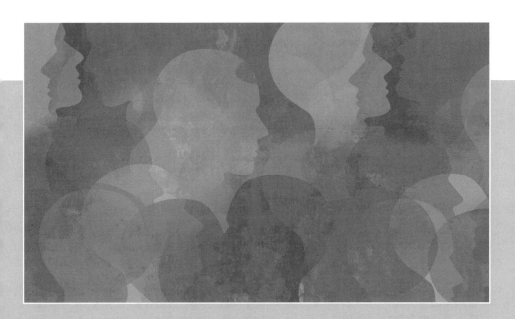

RICHARD RIEGELMAN, MD, MPH, PhD

Professor of Epidemiology, Medicine, and Health Policy, and Founding Dean
The George Washington University Milken Institute School of Public Health
Washington D.C.

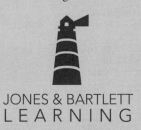

JONES & BARTLETT
LEARNING

World Headquarters
Jones & Bartlett Learning
5 Wall Street
Burlington, MA 01803
978-443-5000
info@jblearning.com
www.jblearning.com

Jones & Bartlett Learning books and products are available through most bookstores and online booksellers. To contact Jones & Bartlett Learning directly, call 800-832-0034, fax 978-443-8000, or visit our website, www.jblearning.com.

Substantial discounts on bulk quantities of Jones & Bartlett Learning publications are available to corporations, professional associations, and other qualified organizations. For details and specific discount information, contact the special sales department at Jones & Bartlett Learning via the above contact information or send an email to specialsales@jblearning.com.

Production Credits
VP, Product Management A&P: Amanda Martin
Director of Product Management: Cathy Esperti
Product Manager: Sophie Fleck Teague
Product Specialist: Carter McAlister
Product Assistant: Tess Sackmann
Director of Production: Jenny L. Corriveau
Director, Relationship Management: Carolyn Rogers Pershouse
Project Manager: Kristen Rogers
Director of Marketing: Andrea DeFronzo
Senior Marketing Manager: Susanne Walker
Production Services Manager: Colleen Lamy
Manufacturing and Inventory Control Supervisor: Amy Bacus
Composition and Project Management: codeMantra U.S. LLC
Cover Design: Kristin E. Parker
Text Design: Kristin E. Parker
Director, Content Services and Licensing: Joanna Gallant
Rights & Media Manager: Shannon Sheehan
Relationship Manager: Merideth Tumasz
Cover Image (Title Page, Chapter Opener): © wildpixel/iStock/Getty Images Plus /Getty Images
Printing and Binding: McNaughton & Gunn
Cover Printing: McNaughton & Gunn

Library of Congress Cataloging-in-Publication Data
Names: Riegelman, Richard K., author.
Title: Population health: a primer / Richard Riegelman.
Description: Burlington, Massachusetts: Jones & Bartlett Learning, [2020] | Includes bibliographical references and index.
Identifiers: LCCN 2018049424 | ISBN 9781284152227 (paperback: alk. paper)
Subjects: | MESH: Population Health | Public Health
Classification: LCC RA418 | NLM WA 300.1 | DDC 362.1—dc23
LC record available at https://lccn.loc.gov/2018049424

6048

Printed in the United States of America
23 22 21 20 19   10 9 8 7 6 5 4 3 2

Contents

Acknowledgments

Brenda Kirkwood, MPH, DrPH, made indispensable contributions to the quality of *Population Health: A Primer* by her careful review, feedback, and editing. J. Zoe Beckerman, MPH, JD, contributed analysis and ideas that are an important part of the text. I would also like to acknowledge the support and encouragement of Mike Brown and his colleagues at Jones & Bartlett Learning who have made a commitment to population health and my ongoing efforts to develop a comprehensive set of materials to lay the foundations for population health education.

Introduction—It Takes a Community to Improve the Population's Health

We have made dramatic progress in improving our population's health over the last dozen decades. A child born in 1900 in the United States was expected to live less than 50 years compared to approximately 80 years today. In 1900, newborns had a 10% chance of dying in the first year of life, and their mothers often died in childbirth. In recent decades, we have reduced the death rate from coronary artery disease by half, cut smoking rates by 50%, and dramatically reduced the deaths from motor vehicle injuries per mile traveled.

Despite the enormous progress we have made, we continue to face new health challenges. The progress we have made has been interrupted at times by widespread occurrence of disease in the form of epidemics and worldwide pandemics. The number of deaths from Influenza A is rivaled only by war and HIV. In recent years, we have seen life expectancy begin to shorten. Obesity, opioid addiction, and antibiotic resistance are among the challenges that are currently threatening our progress in improving the population's health. In addition, the enormous and rising costs of healthcare services now require us to address the associated financial issues.

Responding to these and other emerging threats requires more than clinical health care; it requires a concerted and coordinated effort by the public health system, the healthcare system, and society at large. Putting these pieces together to improve the health of the population is what we mean by population health.

FIGURE INTRO-1 displays what we will call the three pillars of population health and how they need to work together to improve the health of the population.

Population health is rapidly becoming the overarching umbrella for concepts used to integrate the efforts of traditional public health, clinical health care, and public policy interventions into health systems. Population health builds on the methods of health care, traditional public health, and/or public policy interventions to improve the population's health.

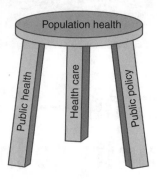

FIGURE INTRO-1 Three Pillars of Population Health

Health care includes the delivery of services to individuals on a one-on-one basis. It includes services for those who are sick or disabled with illness or diseases as well as for those who are asymptomatic. Traditional public health efforts have a population/community-based prevention perspective utilizing interventions targeting populations or communities as well as defined high-risk or vulnerable groups. Communicable disease control, reduction of environmental hazards, food and drug safety, and nutritional and behavioral risk factors have been key areas of focus of traditional public health approaches.

Both health care and traditional public health approaches share a goal to directly affect the health of those they reach. In contrast, public policy interventions can be primarily aimed at nonhealth goals or primarily at affecting health. Public policy interventions range from improving housing, education, transportation, or economic development to providing opportunities for work. They also include efforts to expand and improve Medicare, Medicaid, and other health programs. These various interventions may have dramatic and sometimes unanticipated positive or negative health impacts. Public policy interventions, such as increasing availability of high-quality food, may improve health, while the availability of convenient high-fat or high-calorie foods may pose a risk to health.

TABLE INTRO-1 describes the three pillars of population health, i.e., health care, traditional public health, and public policy, with examples of each.

▶ Why Is Population Health Important?

Population health is key to addressing many of the most difficult health problems we face, from opioid addiction to antibiotic resistance, from emerging infectious diseases to the cost of health care. Population health considers the full range of options for intervention to address these types of complex health problems, from community control of communicable disease and environmental health, to control of the costs of health care, to public policies, such as taxation and laws aimed at reducing cigarette smoking.

No one clinician or healthcare institution can contend with these problems working alone. We need to bring to bear the methods of health care, traditional public health, and/or public policy interventions to improve the population's health.

TABLE INTRO-1 The Three Pillars of Population Health		
	Characteristics	**Examples**
Health care	Systems for delivering one-on-one individual health services, including those aimed at prevention, cure, palliation, and rehabilitation	Clinical preventive services, including vaccinations, behavioral counseling, screening for disease, and preventive medications
Traditional public health	Group- and community-based interventions directed at health promotion and disease prevention	Communicable disease control, control of environmental hazards, food and drug safety, reduction in **risk factors** for disease
Public policy	Interventions with another nonhealth-related purpose that have secondary impacts on health	Interventions that increase access to health services or education, alter nutrition, or address socioeconomic disparities through changes in tax laws

Population health is more than the contribution of each of the pillars of population health. It requires us to understand and utilize three foundational frameworks for thinking. We will categorize these frameworks as follows:

- The Population Health Perspective
- Systems-Thinking and Systems-Doing
- Population Health Tools for Implementation

These foundational frameworks will be the focus of each of the three units of this Primer.

Unit 1—*The Population Health Perspective* will examine the components of population health, the determinants of health and disease, how we measure the course of disease in a population, as well as the health status of a population. We will then examine the basic strategies for improving population health, including when to intervene, how to intervene, and at whom to direct the intervention.

Unit 2—*Systems-Thinking and Systems-Doing* will examine what we mean by systems in general and the health system in particular. We will see how to use systems-thinking to better understand health problems. We will then look at how coordination across professions is central to using systems-thinking to improve the health of the population.

Unit 3—*Population Health Tools for Implementation* will examine the tools of population interventions built on evidence that complements the approaches often used in clinical medicine. These include population-based behavioral change, health communication by mass media and social networking, health policy interventions, **screening** for disease, and population-based **vaccination**.

Each unit will be accompanied by case studies and exercises that illustrate the key concepts and approaches. Boxes will be used to provide more in-depth discussion of important principles and applications.

Population health is a big and important topic that is increasingly expected as part of accredited health professions programs and tested as part of standardized examinations in the health professions.

To begin, let's see what a population health perspective looks like as we start with a short history of HIV/AIDS.

HIV/AIDS: A Population Health History

A report appeared in the Centers for Disease Control and Prevention's "Morbidity and Mortality Weekly Report" (MMWR) on June 5, 1981, describing a previously unknown deadly disease in five young homosexual males, all in Los Angeles. The disease was characterized by dramatically reduced immunity, allowing otherwise innocuous organisms to become "opportunistic infections," rapidly producing fatal infections or cancer. Thus, acquired immunodeficiency syndrome (AIDS) first became known to the public health and medical communities. It was later recognized that HIV did not suddenly appear out of the blue but had a reservoir in primates in Africa and in earlier years had "spilled over" into humans as an emerging infectious disease.

Studies soon associated AIDS with rectal intercourse, blood transfusions, and reuse of injection needles as methods of transmission. Reuse of needles was a common practice in poor nations. It was also widespread among intravenous drug abusers. As a blood-borne disease, concern was raised that it could be transmitted by mosquitoes, but fortunately, there has been no evidence of vectorborne transmission. Within several years, the disease was traced to a previously unknown retrovirus, which came to be called the human immunodeficiency virus (HIV). Studies found that nearly everyone was susceptible to HIV, though a very small percentage of the population had a degree of protection based on their genes.

A test was developed to detect the disease and was first used in testing blood for transfusion. Within a short period of time, the blood supply was protected by testing all donated blood, and transmission of HIV by blood transfusion became a rare event. Diagnostic tests for HIV/AIDS soon became available for testing individuals. For many years, these tests were used by clinicians only for high-risk individuals. In recent years, HIV testing has become more widely used, as the testing no longer requires blood drawing and the results are rapidly available. The Centers for Disease Control and Prevention (CDC) has put increasing emphasis on testing as part of routine health care.

HIV-positive patients were shown to be vulnerable to a large number of opportunistic infections that took advantage of the patient's immune compromised state. From a public health perspective, tuberculosis was especially concerning because of its potential for person-to-person spread. Efforts to control tuberculosis have also led to better control of HIV/AIDS.

Much has been learned about HIV/AIDS. Today, it is primarily a heterosexually transmitted disease with greater risk of transmission from male to females than from females to males. In the United States, African Americans are at the greatest risk. Condoms have been demonstrated to reduce the risk of transmission. Abstinence and monogamous sexual relationships likewise eliminate or greatly reduce the risk. Even serial monogamy reduces the risk compared to multiple simultaneous partners. Male circumcision has been shown to reduce the potential for males to acquire HIV infection by approximately 50%.

In major U.S. cities, the frequency of HIV is often greater than 1% of the population, fulfilling the CDC definition of "high risk." In these geographic areas, the risk of unprotected intercourse is substantially greater than in most suburban or rural areas. Free distribution of condoms in these areas has been widely used. Efforts to reduce high-risk practices, ranging from unprotected anal intercourse to reuse of needles for drug injections, have been tried with some success among high-risk groups.

Maternal-to-child transmission was quite frequent and has been shown to be largely preventable by treatments during pregnancy and at the time of delivery. CDC recommendations for universal HIV testing of pregnant women and intervention for all HIV-positive patients have been widely implemented by clinicians and hospitals and have resulted in greatly reduced or eliminated maternal-to-child transmissions in developed countries and increasingly in developing countries as well.

Medications are now available that greatly reduce the load of HIV present in the blood often to undetectable levels. These medications delay the progression of HIV and reduce the ease of spread of the disease. These treatments were rapidly applied to HIV/AIDS patients in developed countries and eventually in developing countries.

The social stigma attached to HIV/AIDS has gradually, but not completely, disappeared as high-quality health information about HIV/AIDS became widely available. Healthcare organizations and public health organizations shared information on HIV and developed joint plans for efforts, such as eliminating maternal–child transmission and HIV testing. Federal legislation has ensured coverage for HIV care. HIV is increasingly being seen as a chronic manageable disease.

New and emerging approaches to HIV prevention include use of antiviral medications during breastfeeding as well as pre- and postcoital treatment. The lack of availability of testing during the first weeks of infection when HIV is highly transmissible remains a barrier to effective control of HIV. Despite considerable research and some progress, an HIV vaccine still looks like a distant hope for greatly increasing the effectiveness of HIV control efforts. With continued efforts and continued progress, we can look at a future in which HIV/AIDS can be controlled, if not eradicated.

HIV/AIDS addresses many of the population health issues that we will consider in Population Health: A Primer. We will come back to HIV/AIDS after each unit to examine how we can apply the skills of population health to this important population health problem.

In Unit 1, we will examine the determinants of disease and the type of interventions that can be used for prevention, early detection, and treatment of a disease such as HIV/AIDS. In Unit 2, we will look at how we can take a systems approach to understanding a disease such as HIV/AIDS and an approach to addressing disease, which we will call "systems-doing." In Unit 3, we will take a look at the strategies of population health as well as the unique population health tools available to help us reduce the impact of diseases such as HIV/AIDS.

So, let's start in Unit 1 by examining the methods and strategies used in population health using the example of obesity.

UNIT 1

The Population Health Perspective

LEARNING OBJECTIVES

By the end of this unit, students will be able to:

- Define population health and its components
- Describe unique features of population health
- Discuss determinants of health and disease
- Describe measures that are used to quantify population health status
- Discuss options for intervention to improve population health

Obesity is an attribute of individuals, but it can be seen as a population health problem as well as an individual problem. Not only does obesity lead to diabetes and cardiovascular disease, it also has impacts on arthritis and a wide range of muscular-skeletal problems, endocrine, and even liver problems. From the population perspective, obesity is a major cause of death and disability rivaled only by tobacco. Obesity is an attribute of individuals, but addressing the U.S. problem of obesity cannot be dealt with solely by treating one individual at a time. We also need to take a population health approach.

▶ What Are the Components That Comprise Population Health?

Population health examines the health outcomes of groups of individuals, called populations, including the impact of health issues that affect the entire society as well as the health issues of vulnerable or high-risk groups.*

---

* Population health has been defined as "The health outcomes of a group of individuals, including the distribution of such outcomes within the group." These basic concepts are incorporated into the above definition.[1]

To understand population health, we need to describe what we mean by the four components included in this definition:

- Population
- Health
- Health issues affecting the entire society
- Health issues affecting vulnerable groups

▶ What Do We Mean by Population?

The term "**population**" has traditionally referred to individuals living in a geographic area. Today, it is used as a term referring to a defined group of people. Population has come to mean quite different things. There are three basic ways to think of a population:

- Geographically defined population, such as a county, state, or country
- Population defined by a common characteristic, such as membership in a health plan
- Population defined by a common risk factor, such as smoking, chronic pain, or a low socioeconomic group

Therefore, there are three different, but complementary, ways to look at the population component of population health. All of them can be used when speaking of a population. Therefore, it is essential that we understand the way the term "population" is being used in a specific context.

Let's turn back to our example of obesity viewed through the lens of populations.

Obesity and Population

Obesity may be referred to as a population problem. The "population" may refer to a city, state, or country with a high proportion of obesity, such as the 1/3 of U.S. adults who have a body mass index (BMI) of 30 or higher and are therefore considered obese. It could also be the membership of a health plan or another organized group. Finally, the population referred to in population health might be a high-risk group, such as overweight children or those from a low socioeconomic group. Any of these groups may be defined as a population and their problems addressed as part of population health.

▶ What Do We Mean by Health?

For many years, **health** was defined as the absence of disease. In recent years, health has come to mean "A state of complete physical, social and mental well-being, and not merely the absence of disease or infirmity" as defined by the World Health Organization.[2]

Until recently, the concept of health focused almost entirely on physical health. Mental health has now been recognized as an important part of the definition. Conditions such as depression and substance abuse make enormous contributions to disability in populations throughout the world. The boundaries of what we mean by "health" continue to expand, and the limits of health are not clear. Many novel medical interventions—including modification of genes and treatments to increase height, improve cosmetic appearance, and improve sexual or intellectual performance—confront us with this question: are these health issues?

Obesity and Health

Obesity is not itself a disease; it is primarily a risk factor for disease; therefore, obesity has not been an intrinsic aspect of health until recently. Extending the definition of health to include the absence of obesity is a population health approach. Taking a population health approach leads us to consider not only the disease implications of obesity, but also the social implications of obesity, ranging from health insurance coverage for prevention and treatments to the implications for schools, the military, airlines, and many other settings not traditionally thought of as playing a role in health.

The definition of population health requires more than defining what we mean by "population" and "health." It also requires us to consider the implications of health issues affecting the entire society as well as the health issues of vulnerable or high-risk groups.

▶ What Do We Mean by Health Issues Affecting the Entire Society?

Society-wide population health issues have focused and continue to focus on issues such as communicable disease as well as the quality of the air, water, and food that we all share. In recent decades, the focus of society-wide concerns has greatly expanded to include a range of issues, from transportation safety to the costs of health care. Additional population health concerns, ranging from the impact of climate change to the harms and benefits of new technologies, are altering the meaning of society-wide concerns.

Obesity as a Society-Wide Health Issue

The percentage of the U.S. population with obesity has more than doubled in the last half century. Economic and cultural factors have had population-wide impacts on obesity. The introduction of high-fructose corn syrup into a wide range of foods and the rapid growth of the fast food industry have been strongly associated with the development of obesity. The size of the American plate has literally increased. Changes in economics and culture leading to a sedentary lifestyle have contributed to the obesity **epidemic**. Thus, obesity is affected by the result of social forces, not just individual behavior. Interventions to address obesity need to be directed not only at the individual with obesity, but also at the underlying social and economic changes that have played important roles in the increase in obesity.

▶ What Do We Mean by Health Issues Affecting Vulnerable or High-Risk Groups?

Population health focuses not only on society-wide health issues, but also on health issues that affect high-risk subgroups within the society, often called high-risk groups. For most of the 20th century, the focus on vulnerable groups centered on maternal and child health and individuals in high-risk occupations. While these groups remain important, under the umbrella of population health, additional groups now receive increased attention, including the disabled, the frail elderly, and those without health insurance. Attention is also being focused on the immunosuppressed, especially those living with HIV/AIDS, who are at higher risk of infection and illness, and those whose genetic code leads to a special vulnerability to disease and adverse reactions to medications.

Obesity and Vulnerable Groups

Obesity is not uniformly distributed in our society. Lower socioeconomic groups and adults who were sedentary and obese as children are at high risk of being obese as adults. Population health interventions need to be specifically targeted at high risk vulnerable groups as well as at obese individuals and the population as a whole.

▶ What Are the Unique Features of Population Health?

Population health is a broad and changing field, which may look quite different depending on where you stand and the perspective you take. It is important to recognize that population health has a number of unique features. **BOX 1-1** addresses the unique features of population health that distinguish it from individual health care and public health.

BOX 1-1 Unique Features of Population Health

Population health can be seen as a way of thinking that is parallel to the way of thinking used in individual health care. In individual health care, we do the following:

- Describe an individual's problem, including their symptoms and risks for disease
- Make a diagnosis of their diseases or conditions
- Select individual intervention(s) or treatment(s) tailored to the individual's situation and desires.

In population health, there is a parallel way of thinking that requires different approaches from those of clinical medicine. In population health, we do the following:

- Describe a population's problem, including the underlying determinants of health and disease
- Make a diagnosis of the problem using a systems approach
- Select intervention(s) utilizing a wide range of available individual, group, and population-based options for intervention.

Many public health professionals see population health as a natural extension of public health given the long-standing focus of public health on the health of the public and on vulnerable groups. Traditional governmental public health, however, differs from the current approaches to population health in a number of ways:

- Population health explicitly and actively engages the public health system, the healthcare system, as well as public policy efforts that address what we will call the **determinants of health**.
- Population health utilizes what we will call **interventions** designed to improve health outcomes, including reducing death and disability. Interventions include the full spectrum of available options, from prevention to treatment to rehabilitation and palliation.
- Population health takes what we will call a systems approach, which actively looks for effective points to intervene through the public health system, the healthcare system, or through social interventions or policy solutions.
- Population health looks at outcomes rather than organizations. That is, it is focused on the needs of the population, whether these can be best accomplished through hospitals, home care, hospice, or health department services. Population health's outcomes include but are not limited to the prevention of disease plus promotion and protection of health. Cure, rehabilitation, and palliation may also be goals of population health.

Therefore, population health uses a wide range of interventions to improve health outcomes.

Population health science is beginning to emerge to underpin the efforts of population health. Population health science uses health care and public health research and also the research in a wide range of other professions and disciplines, ranging from economics to psychology and from systems analysis to communications.

The focus of population health science includes understanding factors, often called **influences** or determinants, which affect the development and the outcome of disease. Let's take a look at what is meant by the determinants of health.[†]

[†] The term determinants of health has become standard terminology even though no one determinant guarantees an outcome. The term "influences," which as we will see is used in systems analysis, is often a more accurate description since factors such as genes or risk factor exposures may increase the probability of disease but do not determine its occurrence. Since the term "determinants" has become widely used, it will be used here with the understanding that determinants influence but do not determine in-and-of-themselves the outcomes of interest

▶ What Are the Determinants of Health and Disease?

Population health science requires that we first establish **etiology** and **efficacy**. Etiology addresses the contributory cause(s) of disease, while efficacy looks at how interventions can impact the outcome of disease.

Population health, however, frequently goes beyond the immediate causes of disease and the individual interventions that improve outcome. It often looks at the underlying influences or determinants. These determinants have been called "causes of causes."

Thus, determinants look beyond the known contributory causes of disease to factors that are at work often years before a disease develops.[3,4]

These underlying factors may be thought of as "upstream" forces. Like great storms, we know the water will flow downstream, often producing flooding and destruction along the way. We just do not know exactly when and where the destruction will occur. For example, we know that obesity poses risks to health but may not be able to predict whether it will produce arthritis, heart disease, diabetes, liver disease, or a combination. There is no official list or agreed-upon definition of what is included in determinants of disease.[‡]

Nonetheless, there is wide agreement that the following factors are among those that can be described as determinants of health in that they increase or at times decrease the chances of developing conditions that threaten the quantity and/or quality of life. Some but not all of these factors are related to socioeconomic-cultural factors and are categorized as **social determinants of health**.

Behavior

Infection

Genetics

Geography

Environment

Medical care

Socioeconomic-cultural

The mnemonic **BIG GEMS** provides a convenient device for remembering these determinants of disease. Let's see what we mean by each of the determinants.

Behavior: This implies actions that increase exposure to the factors that produce disease or protect individuals from disease. Actions such as smoking cigarettes,

---

‡ Health Canada has identified 12 determinants of health, which are (1) income and social status, (2) employment, (3) education, (4) social environments, (5) physical environments, (6) healthy child development, (7) personal health practices and coping skills, (8) health services, (9) social support networks, (10) biology and genetic endowment, (11) gender, and (12) culture. Many of these are subsumed under socioeconomic-cultural determinants in the BIG GEMS framework. The World Health Organization's Commission on Social Determinants of Health has also produced a list of determinants that is consistent with the BIG GEMS framework.[3,4]

exercising, eating a particular diet, consuming alcohol, having an influenza vaccine, having unprotected intercourse, and using seat belts are all examples of the ways in which behaviors help determine the development of disease.

Infections: These are often the direct cause of disease. In addition, we are increasingly recognizing that early or long-standing exposures to infections may contribute to the development of disease or even protection against disease. Diseases as diverse as gastric and duodenal ulcers, gallstones, and hepatoma are increasingly thought to have infection as an important determinant. Early exposure to infections may actually reduce diseases ranging from polio to asthma through their impact on the microbial environment in our gastrointestinal tract, increasingly referred to as our **human microbiome**.

Genetics: The revolution in genetics has focused our attention on roles that genetic factors play in the development and outcome of disease. Even when contributory causes, such as cigarettes, have been clearly established as producing lung cancer, genetic factors also play a role in the development and progression of the disease. While genetic factors play a role in many diseases as well as the outcome of disease, they are only occasionally the most important determinant of disease.

Geography: Geographic location influences the frequency and even the presence of disease. Infectious diseases, such as malaria, Zika, Chagas disease, schistosomiasis, and Lyme disease, occur only in defined geographic areas. Geography may also imply local geological conditions, such as those that produce high levels of radon—a naturally occurring radiation that contributes to the development of lung cancer. Geography also implies that features of special locations can produce disease, such as altitude sickness in high elevations, frostbite in cold climates, or certain types of snake bites in the tropics.

Environment: Environmental factors determine disease and the course of disease in a number of ways. The **unaltered environment** or "natural" physical world around us may produce disability and death from sudden natural disasters, such as earthquakes and volcanic eruptions to iodine deficiencies due to low iodine content in the food-producing soil. The **altered environment**, which we often call pollution, produced by human intervention includes exposures to toxic substances in occupational or nonoccupational settings. Finally, the physical environment includes the environment built for use by humans—the **built environment**—which produces determinants ranging from indoor air pollution to "infant-proofed" homes to hazards on the highway.

Medical care: Access to and the quality of medical care can be a determinant of disease. When a high percentage of individuals is protected by vaccination, nonvaccinated individuals in the population may be protected as well. Cigarette smoking cessation efforts may help smokers quit, and treatment for infectious disease may reduce the spread to others. Medical care, however, often has its major impact on the course of disease by attempting to prevent or minimize disability and death once disease develops.

Socioeconomic-cultural: In the United States, socioeconomic factors have been defined as education, income, and occupational status. These measures have all been shown to be determinants for diseases as varied as breast cancer, tuberculosis (TB), and occupational injuries. Cultural and religious factors are increasingly being recognized as determinants of the development of disease. In addition, because beliefs or cultural habits may influence decisions about treatments, these in turn may affect the outcome of the disease. While most diseases occur in lower socioeconomic groups more frequently, others, such as breast cancer or food allergies, may be more common in higher socioeconomic groups.

In **BOX 1-2,** let's take a look at an example of how the BIG GEMS mnemonic can be used to identify potential determinants of a disease.

BOX 1-2 Asthma and the Determinants of Disease

Let's look at determinants of disease with a traditional clinical case study using an individual patient.

Jennifer, a teenager living in a rundown urban apartment in a city with high levels of air pollution, develops severe asthma. Her mother also has severe asthma, yet both of them smoke cigarettes. Her clinician prescribed medications to prevent asthma attacks, but she takes them only when she experiences severe symptoms. Jennifer is hospitalized twice with pneumonia due to common bacterial infections. She then develops an antibiotic-resistant infection. During this hospitalization, she requires intensive care on a respirator. After several weeks of intensive care and every known treatment to save her life, she dies suddenly.

Asthma is an inflammatory disease of the lung coupled with an increased reactivity of the airways, which together produce a narrowing of the airways of the lungs. When the airways become swollen and inflamed, they become narrower, allowing less air through to the lung tissue and causing symptoms such as wheezing, coughing, chest tightness, breathing difficulty, and predisposition to infection. Once considered a minor ailment, asthma is now the most common chronic disorder of childhood. It affects over 6 million children under the age of 18 in the United States alone.

Jennifer's tragic history illustrates how a wide range of determinants of disease may affect the occurrence, severity, and development of complications of a disease. Let's walk through the BIG GEMS framework and see how each determinant had an impact on Jennifer.

Behavior: Behavioral factors play an important role in the development of asthma attacks and their complications. Cigarette smoking makes asthma attacks more frequent and more severe. It also predisposes individuals to developing infections such as pneumonia. Treatment for severe asthma requires regular use along with more intensive treatment when an attack occurs. It is difficult for many people, especially teenagers, to take medication regularly, yet failure to adhere to treatment greatly complicates the disease.

Infection: This is a frequent precipitant of asthma, and asthma increases the frequency and severity of infections. Infectious diseases, especially pneumonia, can be life-threatening in asthmatics, requiring prompt and high-quality medical care. The increasing development of antibiotic-resistant infections poses special risks to those with asthma.

Genetics: Genetic factors predispose people to childhood asthma. However, many children and adults without a family history develop asthma.

Geography: Asthma is more common in geographic areas with high levels of naturally occurring allergens due to flowering plants. However, today, even populations in desert climates in the United States are often affected by asthma, as irrigation results in the planting of allergen-producing trees and other plants.

Environment: The physical environment, including that built for use by humans, has increasingly been recognized as a major factor affecting the development of asthma and asthma attacks. Indoor air pollution due to wood burning is the most common form of air pollution in many developing countries. Along with cigarette smoke, air pollution inflames the lungs acutely and chronically. Cockroaches often found in rundown buildings have been found to be highly allergenic and predisposing to asthma. Other factors in the built environment, including mold and exposure to pet dander, can also trigger wheezing in susceptible individuals.

Medical care: The course of asthma can be greatly affected by medical care. Management of the acute and chronic effects of asthma can be positively affected by efforts to understand an individual's exposures, reducing the chronic inflammation with medications, managing the acute symptoms, and avoiding life-threatening complications.

Socioeconomic-cultural: Disease and disease progression are often influenced by an individual's socioeconomic status. Air pollution is often greater in lower socioeconomic neighborhoods of urban areas. Mold and cockroach infestations may be greater in poor neighborhoods with poorly maintained buildings. Access to and quality of medical care may be affected by social, economic, and cultural factors.

Asthma is a condition that demonstrates the contributions made by the full range of determinants included in the BIG GEMS framework. No one determinant alone explains the bulk of the disease. The large number of determinants and their interactions provide opportunities for a **population health approach** using health care, traditional public health, and public policy interventions.

▶ What Changes in Populations Over Time Can Affect Health?

A number of important trends or transitions in the size and composition of populations that affect the pattern of disease have been described in recent years. These transitions have implications for what we can expect to happen throughout the 21st century. We will call these the demographic and epidemiological transitions.

The **demographic transition** describes the impacts of falling childhood death rates and extended life spans on the size and age distribution of populations.[5] During the first half of the 20th century, death rates among the young fell dramatically in today's developed countries. Death rates continued their dramatic decline in most parts of the developing world during the second half of the 20th century.

Birth rates tend to remain high for years or decades after the decline in deaths. High birth rates paired with lower death rates lead to rapid growth in population size, as we have seen in much of the developing world. This trend continues today in some countries and is expected to go on in some parts of the world well into the 21st century.

Population pyramids are often useful for displaying changes in age distribution that occur over time. Population pyramids display the number of males and the number of females that are alive or expected to be alive for each age group in a particular year. The population pyramids in **FIGURE 1-1** illustrate how the population of Nigeria is expected to grow through 2050 due to a high birth rate and a lowered death rate.[5]

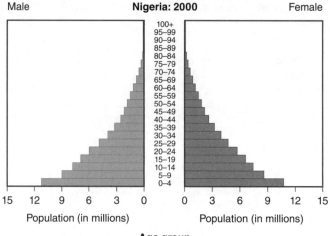

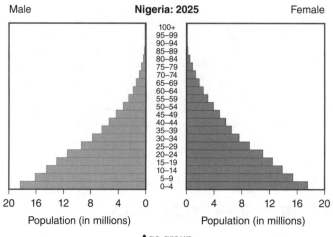

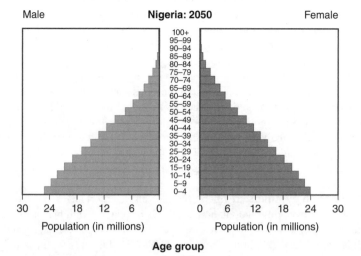

FIGURE 1-1 Population Pyramid Expected for Nigeria

Reproduced from U.S. Census Bureau. International Database. Available at https://www.census.gov/data-tools/demo/idb/informationGateway.php. Accessed July 16, 2018.

Despite a delay, the decline in birth rates reliably occurs following the decline in childhood deaths. This decline in births gradually leads to aging of the population and can eventually lead to declining population numbers in the absence of large-scale immigration. We are now seeing societies in much of Europe and Japan as well as the United States with rapidly growing elderly populations. Over 25% of the population of Japan is currently over 65 compared to approximately 15% in the United States.

Take a look at the population pyramids in **FIGURE 1-2**, which show what is expected to occur in the coming years in much of Europe and Japan.[5] Japan is used as an example of the emergence of an inverted population pyramid, with a smaller young population and a larger older population. Populations with a large number of elderly relative to the number of younger individuals have a heavier burden of disease and create conditions for aging to become a population health issue.

The large number of young immigrants to the United States and their generally higher birth rates have slowed this process in the United States, but the basic trend of a growing elderly population continues.[5] The population pyramids for the United States are displayed in **FIGURE 1-3**.

A second related transition is called the **epidemiological transition**.[6] The epidemiological or public health transition implies that as social and economic development occurs, different types of diseases become prominent. Deaths in less developed societies are often dominated by epidemic communicable diseases and diseases associated with malnutrition and childhood infections. As a country develops, communicable diseases often come under control, and noncommunicable and chronic diseases, such as heart disease, often predominate. In addition, environmental and safety issues are affected by social economic development as air pollution and transportation safety become important issues.

The shape of the population pyramid and the stage of epidemiological transition are important factors in defining a population's burden of disease and disability since the frequency of specific diseases and conditions differs dramatically by age throughout the life cycle.

The low birth rates and increased longevity seen in many developed countries often lead to a small number of workers supporting a large aging population. It also leads to a healthcare and public health system dominated by chronic and noninfectious diseases, including heart disease, cancer, Alzheimer's, and degenerative diseases. Therefore, it is important to understand what is called a nation's **population dynamics**, along with the determinants of health, to understand the current population health problems and anticipate population health problems in the coming years.

In order to measure the outcomes of population health, we need to have measurements that summarize the health of the population. Let's take a look at the most commonly used measurements.

▶ How Do We Measure the Health of a Population?

Measurements that summarize the health of populations are called **population health status measures**. For over a century, we used measures of the health status of large populations, such as countries and large groups within countries—for

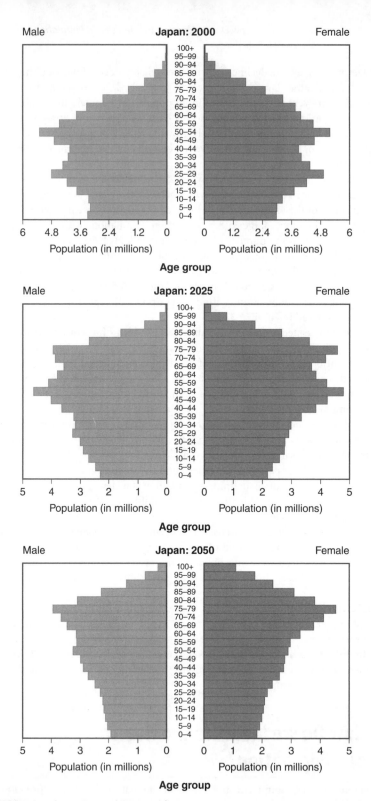

FIGURE 1-2 Population Pyramid Expected for Japan

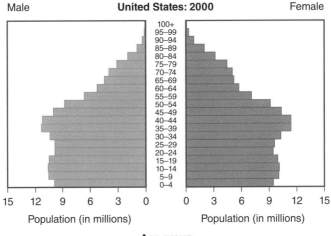

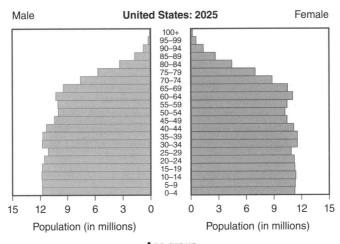

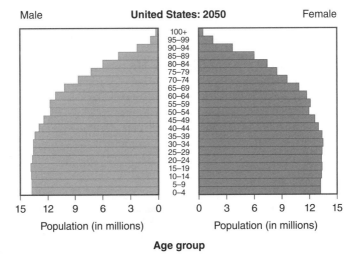

FIGURE 1-3 Population Pyramid Expected for the United States

example, males and females or large racial groups of a particular nation. In the 20th century, two measurements became the standard for summarizing the health status of populations: the **infant mortality rate** and **life expectancy**. These measurements rely on death and birth certificate data as well as census data. Toward the latter part of the 20th century, these sources of data became widely available and quite accurate in most parts of the world.

The infant mortality rate estimates the rate of death in the first year of life per 1000 live births. For many years, it was used as the primary measurement of child health. Life expectancy was used to measure the overall death experience of the population, incorporating the probability of dying in each year of life.[7,8] These measures were the mainstay of 20th-century population health measurements. Let's look at each of these measures and see why additional health status measurements are needed for the 21st century.

In the early years of the 20th century, infant mortality rates were high even in what are today's developed countries, such as the United States. It was not unusual for 100 or even 200 of every 1000 newborns to die in the first year of their lives. In most parts of the world, infant mortality far exceeded the death rate in any later years of childhood. For this reason, the infant mortality rate was often used as a surrogate or substitute measure for overall rates of childhood death. In the first half of the 20th century, however, great improvements in infant mortality occurred in what are today's developed countries. During the second half of the century, many developing countries also saw greatly reduced infant mortality rates. Today, many countries have achieved infant mortality rates below 10 per 1000 live births, and a growing number of nations have achieved rates below 5 per 1000.[§]

The degree of success in reducing mortality among children aged 2–5 has not been as great.[9] Malnutrition and old and new infectious diseases continue to kill young children. In addition, improvements in the care of severely ill newborns have extended the lives of many children—only to have them die after the first year of their life. Children with HIV/AIDS often die not in the first year of life, but in the second, third, or fourth year. Once a child survives to age 5, he or she has a very high probability of surviving into adulthood in most countries. Thus, a new measurement known as **under-5 mortality** has now become the standard health status measure used by the World Health Organization (WHO) to summarize the health of children.

Let's take a look at the second traditional measure of population health status: life expectancy. Life expectancy is a snapshot of a population incorporating the probability of dying at each age of life in a particular year. Life expectancy tells us how well a country is doing in terms of deaths in a particular year. As an example, current life expectancy at birth in a developed country may be 80 years. Perhaps in 1900, life expectancy at birth in that same country was only

---

§ The infant mortality rate is measured using the number of deaths among those in the ages 0–1 in a particular year divided by the total number of live births in the same year. If the number of live births is stable from year to year, then the infant mortality rate is a measure of the incidence rate of deaths. Health status measurements of child health have not sought to incorporate disability on the less-than-completely-accurate assumption that disability is not a major factor among children.

50 years. In a few countries, life expectancy at birth for women already exceeds 85 years. Thus, life expectancy allows us to make comparisons between countries, compare large groups such as males and females within a country, and measure changes over time.

Life expectancy can be calculated at any age, so we may speak of life expectancy at age 65 or age 85. Despite its name, life expectancy cannot be used to accurately predict an individual's future life span or even the life span of a population. Prediction requires assuming that nothing will change. That is, accurate prediction requires the death rates at all ages to remain the same in future years. We have seen increases in life expectancy in most countries over the last century, but declines occurred in sub-Saharan Africa and countries of the former Soviet Union in the late 20th century.⁋

Under-5 mortality and life expectancy address only death or **mortality**; they do not incorporate **morbidity** or quality of health. Population health measures need to address issues of quality as well as length of life.

▶ How Can We Incorporate the Quality of Health into Population Health Measures?

Life expectancy tells us only part of what we want to know. It reflects the impact of dying, but not the impact of disabilities. When considering the health status of a population in the 21st century, we need to consider disability as well as death.

Today, the WHO uses a measurement known as the **health-adjusted life expectancy (HALE)** to summarize the health of populations.[10] The measurement of HALE starts with life expectancy and then incorporates measurements of the quality of health. WHO utilizes survey data to obtain a country's overall measurement of quality of health. This measurement incorporates key components, including the following:**

- Mobility: The ability to walk without assistance
- Cognition: Mental function, including memory
- Self-care: Activities of daily living, including dressing, eating, bathing, and use of the toilet
- Pain: Regular pain that limits function
- Mood: Alteration in mood that limits function
- Sensory organ function: Impairment in vision or hearing that impairs function

---

⁋ Life expectancy is greater than you may expect at older ages. For instance, in a country with a life expectancy of 80 years, a 60-year-old may still have a life expectancy of 25 years, not 20 years, because he or she escaped the risks of death during the early years of life. At age 80, the chances of death are very dependent on an individual's state of health because life expectancy combines the probability of death of those in good health and those in poor health. Healthy 80-year-olds have a very high probability of living to 90 and beyond.

** It can be argued that use of these measurements associate disability primarily with the elderly. Note that these qualities of health do not specifically include measures of the ability to work, engage in social interactions, or have satisfying sexual relationships, all of which may be especially important to younger populations.

A quality of health measurement of 90% for a country indicates that the average person in the country loses 10% of his or her full health over his or her lifetime to one or more disabilities. In most countries, the quality of health ranges from 85% to 90%. We might consider a score of less than 85% poor and greater than 90% very good.

The quality of health measurement is multiplied by the life expectancy at birth to obtain the HALE. Thus, a country that has achieved a life expectancy at birth of 80 years and an overall quality of health score of 90% can claim a HALE of $80.00 \times 0.90 = 72.00$.

TABLE 1-1 displays WHO data on life expectancy at birth and HALEs[10] for a variety of large countries.[††]

TABLE 1-1 Life Expectancy and Health-Adjusted Life Expectancy for a Range of Large Countries		
Country	**Life expectancy**	**Health-adjusted life expectancy (HALE)**
Nigeria	54.5	47.4
India	68.3	59.5
Brazil	75.0	65.5
China	76.1	68.5
United States	79.3	69.1
United Kingdom	81.2	71.4
Canada	82.2	72.3
Japan	83.7	74.9

Data from World Health Organization. Healthy life expectancy (HLE) at birth (years). World Health Statistics 2016. http://www.who.int/gho/publications/world_health_statistics/2016/en/ Accessed July 16, 2018.

††In addition to HALE, a measurement known as the **health-related quality of life (HRQOL)** has been developed and used in the United States. HRQOL incorporates a measure of unhealthy days. Unhealthy days are measured by asking a representative sample of individuals the number of days in the last 30 days during which the status of either their mental or physical health kept them from their usual activities. It then calculates a measure of the quality of health by adding together the number of unhealthy days due to mental plus physical health. The quality of health is obtained by dividing the number of healthy days by 30. This measurement is relatively easy to collect and calculate, but unlike HALE, it does not reflect objective measures of disability and cannot be directly combined with life expectancy to produce an overall measure of health. That is, it does not include the impact of mortality.

Today, the under-5 mortality rate and HALE are used by WHO as the standard measures reflecting child health and the overall health of a population.

An additional measure, known as the **disability-adjusted life year (DALY)**, has been developed and used by WHO to allow for comparisons and changes based on specific disease and categories of disease as well as risk factors for disease.[11] DALYs are a measure of the overall disease burden, expressed as the number of years lost due to ill-health, disability, or early death. One DALY can be thought of as the loss of 1 year of life at full health for one individual. **BOX 1-3** describes DALYs.

We have now looked at ways in which we can measure population health status. In addition to summarizing the health of populations, population health requires that we examine the potential for disease to spread in a population.

▶ How Do We Measure the Potential for Spread of a Disease?

We would like to be able to understand the potential for spread of disease to others. The concept of spread of disease is traditionally thought of in terms of communicable

---

BOX 1-3 DALYs

DALYs are designed to examine the impacts that specific diseases and risk factors have on populations as well as to provide an overall measure of population health status. They allow comparisons between countries or within countries over time based not only on overall summary numbers, such as life expectancy and HALEs, but also on specific diseases and risk factors.

DALY compares a country's performance to the country with the longest life expectancy, which is currently Japan. Japan has a life expectancy, for men and women combined, of approximately 83 years. In a country with zero DALYs, the average person would live approximately 83 years without any disability and would then die suddenly. Of course, this does not occur even in Japan, so all countries have DALYs of greater than zero. The measurement is usually presented as DALYs per 1000 population in a particular country.*

Calculations of DALYs require much more data on specific diseases and disabilities than other measurements, such as life expectancy or HALEs. However, WHO's Global Burden of Disease (GBD) project has made considerable progress in obtaining worldwide data collected using a consistent approach.[11] Data on the disability produced by a disease are often not available. WHO then uses expert opinion to estimate the impact.

---

* The newest version of the WHO DALY measurement differs from the previous versions and the numbers should not be compared. Prevalence and not incidence is used in the current version. In addition, WHO no longer discounts DALYs. Interpretation of DALYs can be confusing. If 1000 newborns suddenly died in a country with 0 DALYs, there would be a loss of as much as 83,000 DALYs from the death of these 1000 newborns. Thus, the total DALYs a country can lose in a particular year can range from 0 to approximately 83,000 per 1000 persons. It is possible for a country to have more than 1000 DALYs lost per 1000 population. For instance, WHO reports that Angola has 1046 DALYs per 1000 population. If a country loses 1000 DALYs per 1000 population, it implies that 1 year of healthy life is lost for every year of life lived; that is, half the years of healthy life are lost. Those years of life lost mostly occur in future years since they are based on death and disability over the future life span.

disease. However, as we will see, other types of epidemics, such as the obesity and opioid crisis, can also be thought of as spreading within a population.

R_0 **(R naught)** is the fundamental population health measure of the potential for a disease to spread. It has gained wide visibility through movies and the media as an indication of the potential of a disease to cause an epidemic.

R_0 measures the average number of infections produced by an infected individual exposed to an otherwise entirely susceptible population. If R_0 is less than 1, then the average person with the disease will spread the disease to less than one other person. Therefore, the number of people with disease will decline over time, making the occurrence of an epidemic very unlikely.

On the other hand, if R_0 is greater than 1, an individual with the disease will on average spread it to one or more others, which means that the disease has the potential for becoming an epidemic. The higher the R_0, the more likely the occurrence of an epidemic. Thus, R_0 has been used to estimate the degree of communicability of a disease and the potential of the disease to lead to an epidemic.[12] **TABLE 1-2** provides examples of R_0 that have been calculated for different diseases.

BOX 1-4 looks at how R_0 can be used to estimate the impact of a vaccine as well as the limitation of R_0.

We have now examined what we mean by population health, the factors that influence population health, and how we measure population health as well as the spread of a disease in a population. We are ready to ask what we can do about it. Population health considers a wide range of options for intervention. Let's look at a population health framework for selecting one or more options for intervention to address a health problem.

TABLE 1-2 Examples of Estimated R_0 for Selected Communicable Diseases

Disease	Estimated R_0
Measles	18
Mumps	10
HIV	4
Severe acute respiratory syndrome (SARS)	4
Ebola	2
Hepatitis C	2

Data from Ramirez, VB. What is R_0?: Gauging contagious infections. Healthline. http://www.healthline.com/health/r-nought -reproduction-number#R0values2. Accessed July 16, 2018.

BOX 1-4 Uses and Limitations of R_0

R_0 can be used to estimate the proportion or percentage of a population that needs to be protected by vaccination or other means, such as disease exposure, to prevent the development of an epidemic.[13,14] Protection often requires effective immunizations, so it is important to estimate both the effectiveness of the vaccine and the proportion of the population that is vaccinated. The proportion of the population that needs to be effectively vaccinated is calculated as

$$1 - \frac{1}{R_0}$$

This formula predicts the following:

- When the R_0 is 1.2, an epidemic may be prevented by effective immunization of approximately 17% of the population
- When the R_0 is 1.5, an epidemic may be prevented by effective immunization of approximately 33% of the population
- When the R_0 is 2.0, an epidemic may be prevented by effective immunization of approximately 50% of the population
- When the R_0 is 4.0, an epidemic may be prevented by effective immunization of approximately 75% of the population
- When the R_0 is 10 or higher, an epidemic may be prevented by effective immunization of 90% or more of the population.

This suggests that control of diseases with a large R_0, such as measles and mumps, requires very high levels of effective immunization, which are very difficult to obtain and maintain.

R_0 does not allow us to predict how long it will take for an epidemic to develop, but it can be used alone to predict the proportion or percentage of the population that will eventually be infected if no effective interventions are implemented.

Despite the usefulness of R_0, it is important to recognize its inherent limitations and cautions in its application. Standard estimates of R_0 assume not only that everyone is susceptible to the disease, but also that all individuals have an equal probability of exposure. In diseases such as HIV and hepatitis B, the probability of infections is largely limited to high-risk groups.*

R_0 has become an important measurement in the investigation and control of communicable disease. However, it is important to understand its meaning, uses, and limitations.

---

* R_0 also assumes that there is an average transmission probability. In some diseases, such as SARS, "super spreaders" have been recognized that may infect a large number of individuals and play a disproportionate role in producing an epidemic. In addition, transmission probability may vary throughout the course of a disease. For instance, HIV often has a very high initial probability of transmission followed by much lower levels of transmission once the acute infection is controlled.

▶ What Are the Options for Intervention to Improve Population Health?

Today, there are often a large number of possible interventions to consider when addressing health problems. Many of the interventions have potential harms as well as potential benefits. The large and growing array of possible interventions means that population health decisions require a systematic method for deciding which intervention(s) to use and how to combine them in the most effective and efficient ways. Let's return to our obesity example to outline some of the potential interventions that might be used.

Interventions for Obesity

Obesity might be prevented by increasing physical activity, reducing the use of high-fructose corn syrup, or changing cultural habits that encourage obesity. Early detection and interventions in childhood may lead to reduced adult obesity. Early intervention may also minimize the impacts of obesity on diabetes, other endocrine disorders, as well as muscular skeletal conditions. Interventions aimed at those with long-standing obesity might focus on preventing complications and even on reversal of complications through interventions such as medications and surgery.

A useful framework for examining the options for implementation uses a structure, which we will call the "When–Who–How" approach.

"When" asks about the timing in the course of disease in which an intervention occurs. This timing allows us to categorize interventions as primary, secondary, and tertiary. **Primary interventions** take place before the onset of the disease. They aim to prevent the disease from occurring. **Secondary interventions** occur after the development of a disease or risk factor, but before symptoms appear. They are aimed at early detection of disease or reducing risk factors while the individual is asymptomatic. **Tertiary interventions** occur after the initial occurrence of symptoms, but before irreversible disability. They aim to prevent irreversible consequences of the disease.

For cigarette smoking and lung cancer, primary interventions aim to prevent cigarette smoking. Secondary interventions aim to reverse the course of disease by smoking cessation efforts or screening to detect early disease. Tertiary interventions diagnose and treat diseases caused by smoking in order to prevent permanent disability and death.‡‡

---

‡‡ The CDC defines four levels of intervention: the individual, the relationship (for example, the family), the community, and society or the population as a whole. This framework has the advantage of separating immediate family interventions from community interventions. The group or at-risk group relationship used here may at times refer to the family unit or geographic communities. It may also refer to institutions or at-risk vulnerable groups within the community. The use of group or at-risk group relationships provides greater flexibility, allowing application to a wider range of situations. In addition, the three levels used here correlate with the measurements of relative risk, attributable risk percentage, and population attributable percentage, which are the fundamental epidemiological measurements applied to the magnitude of the impact of an intervention.

"Who" asks: at whom should we direct the intervention? Should it be directed at individuals one at a time as part of clinical care? Alternatively, should it be directed at groups of people, such as vulnerable populations, or should it be directed at everyone in a community or population?

Finally, we need to ask: how should we implement interventions? There are three basic types of interventions when addressing the need for behavioral change. These interventions can be classified as information (education), motivation (incentives), and obligation (requirements).§§

An information or education strategy aims to change behavior through individual encounters, group interactions, or the mass media. Motivation implies use of incentives for changing or maintaining behavior. It implies more than strong or enthusiastic encouragement—it implies tangible reward. Obligation relies on laws and regulations requiring specific behaviors.

TABLE 1-3 outlines how we can combine the "who" and the "how" to develop a series of population health approaches to reduce the risk of cigarettes.

Deciding when, who, and how to intervene depends in a large part upon the available options and the evidence that they work. It also depends in part on our attitudes toward different types of interventions. Some in the United States prefer to rely on informational or educational strategies. These approaches preserve freedom of choice, which we typically value in the United States in public as well as private decisions. Use of mass media informational strategies may be quite economical and efficient and relative to the large number of individuals they reach through messages, but they often need to be tailored to different audiences. However, information is often ineffective in accomplishing behavioral change—at least on its own.

Strategies based upon motivation, such as taxation and other incentives, may at times be more effective than information alone, though educational strategies are still critical to justify and reinforce motivational interventions. Motivational interventions should be carefully constructed and judiciously used, or they may result in what has been called **victim blaming**. For example, victim blaming in the case of cigarette smoking implies that we regard the consequences of smoking as the smokers' own fault.

The use of obligation or legally required action can be quite effective through clear-cut behavior and relatively simple enforcement, such as restrictions on indoor public smoking. These types of efforts may be regarded by some as a last resort, but others may see them as a key to effective use of other strategies. Obligation inevitably removes some freedom of choice. As a result, obligations often have impacts on individual rights, which we hold in high regard in the United States. Enforcement can be expensive as well. Thus, obligation strategies require careful consideration before use as intervention options, as do motivation and education options. Pros and cons of any strategy should be determined after deciding on the clear goals to be accomplished.

We have now looked at the components of population health, including defining the meaning of population, health, health issues affecting the entire society, as

---

§§ An additional option is innovation. Innovation implies a technical or engineering solution. A distinct advantage of technical or engineering solutions is that they often require far less behavior change. Changing human behavior is frequently difficult. Nonetheless, it is an essential component of most, if not all, successful population health interventions. Certainly, that is the case with cigarette smoking.

TABLE 1-3 Examples of "Who" and "How" Related to Cigarette Smoking

	Information	Motivation	Obligation
Individual	Clinician provides patient with information explaining reasons for changing behavior	Clinician encourages patient to change behavior in order to qualify for a service or gain a benefit (e.g., status or financial)	Clinician denies patient a service unless patient changes behavior
	Example: Clinician distributes educational packet to a smoker and discusses his or her own smoking habit	Example: Clinician suggests that the financial savings from not buying cigarettes be used to buy a luxury item	Example: Clinician implements recommendation to refuse birth control pills to women over 35 who smoke cigarettes
High-risk group	Information is made available to all those who engage in a behavior	Those who engage in a behavior are required to pay a higher price	Those who engage in a behavior are barred from an activity or job
	Example: Warning labels on cigarette packages	Example: Taxes on cigarettes	Example: Smokers banned from jobs that will expose them to fumes that may damage their lungs
Population	Information is made available to the entire population, including those who do not engage in the behavior	Incentives are provided for those not at risk to discourage the behavior in those at risk	An activity is required or prohibited for those at risk and also for those not at risk of the condition
	Example: Media information on the dangers of smoking	Example: Lower healthcare costs for everyone results from reduced percentage of smokers	Example: Cigarette sales banned for those under 18

well as health issues affecting vulnerable or high-risk groups. We have also discussed the determinants of health and the health status measures that are used to assess the health of populations as well as the potential for spread of disease in a population. Finally, we looked at the When–Who–How approach to consider options for implementation to improve the health of the population.

The theme that connects the pieces of population health discussed so far is a focus on the health of a population, not just the health of one individual at a time. This focus on the health of the population or a **population perspective** is the first pillar of population health.

A second pillar of population health is what we will call systems-thinking. Systems-thinking incorporates the building blocks we have discussed. It often allows us to come up with population health strategies for implementation, which lead to effective and efficient approaches to health problems. In Unit 2, we will explore what we mean and how we can use systems-thinking as the second pillar of population health.

🔎 CASE STUDIES AND DISCUSSION QUESTIONS

HIV/AIDS: A Population Health History
Return to the HIV/AIDS case study in the introduction and respond to the following questions.

Discussion Questions
1. Use the BIG GEMS framework to outline the determinants of health discussed in this case.
2. What role has health care played in controlling or failing to control the HIV/AIDS epidemic?
3. What role has traditional public health played in controlling or failing to control the HIV/AIDS epidemic?
4. What roles have social factors (beyond the sphere of health care or public health) played in controlling or failing to control the HIV/AIDS epidemic?

José and Jorge: Identical Twins Without Identical Lives
José and Jorge were identical twins separated at birth. José grew up in a large family in an impoverished slum in the middle of a crime-ridden and polluted district of a major city. Jorge grew up in an upper-middle-class professional family with one other brother in a suburban community in the same city. Despite the fact that José and Jorge were identical twins, their lives and health could not have been more different.

José had few opportunities for medical care or public health services as a child. His nutrition was always marginal, and he developed severe cases of diarrhea before he was 1 year of age. He received a polio vaccine as part of a community vaccination program, but never received vaccinations for measles, mumps, rubella,

(continues)

🔍 CASE STUDIES AND DISCUSSION QUESTIONS

(continued)

or other childhood illnesses. At the age of 4, he developed measles and was so sick that his mother was sure he would not make it.

As a child, José also developed asthma, which seemed to worsen when he played outdoors on hot smoggy days. Dropping out of school at age 14, José went to work in a factory, but quit when he found himself panting for breath at the end of the day.

As a teenager, José was repeatedly exposed to crime and drugs. Once he was caught in the cross fire of gangs fighting for control of drugs in his community. Experimenting with drugs with his teenage friends, José contracted HIV from the use of contaminated needles. He did not know he had HIV until he was nearly 30 years old and developed TB. He did receive free-of-charge treatment for TB from the health department, but once he felt better, he did not follow up with the treatment.

By the time his TB returned, José had lost 30 pounds and could barely make it into the emergency room of the public hospital because of his shortness of breath. He was hospitalized for the last 2 months of his life, mostly to prevent others from being exposed to what was now drug-resistant TB. No one ever knew how many people José exposed to HIV or TB.

Jorge's life as a child was far less eventful. He received "well child" care from an early age. His family hardly noticed that he rarely developed diarrhea and had few sick days from diseases of childhood. He did well in school, but like José, he developed asthma. With good treatment, Jorge was able to play on sports teams, at least until he began to smoke cigarettes at age 14.

Jorge soon began to gain weight, and by the time he graduated from college, he was rapidly becoming obese. In his 20s, he developed high blood pressure, and in his 30s, he had early signs of diabetes. Jorge had a heart attack in his mid-40s and underwent bypass surgery a few years later. The treatments for diabetes, hypertension, and high cholesterol worked well, and Jorge was able to lead a productive professional life into his 40s.

By the time Jorge turned 50, his diabetes began to worsen, and he developed progressive kidney disease. He soon needed twice-a-week dialysis, which kept him alive as he awaited a kidney transplant.

Discussion Questions

1. How do social determinants of health contribute to the different disease patterns of José and Jorge?
2. How do factors in the physical environment explain differences in the health of José and Jorge?
3. What role does medical care play in the differences between the health outcomes of José and Jorge?
4. What roles do public health services play in the health outcomes of José and Jorge?

Sharma's Village

Sharma lives in a small farming village in south Asia, but she could just as well be living in Haiti, Ethiopia, Nigeria, or several dozen other countries classified by the World Bank as low-income economies. Her home is a small hut, and she works daily with her mother to gather firewood for their small indoor fireplace, which acts as the kitchen stove. The smoke often makes her eyes water because there is no chimney or other ventilation.

At night, she sleeps with her extended family in a room where mosquitoes bite her regularly. Despite the fact that Sharma lives in a rural community, the villagers live in crowded quarters. The water the family drinks is carried by the women from a well several hundred yards from their home. The water tastes bad sometimes, but it is all they have to drink.

The family farms a small plot of land on the hillside, which had become eroded from years of cutting trees. The last big monsoon to hit the area created a landslide, which left the village underwater for several weeks, creating mold in nearly every home. Most of the adults have goiters from the lack of iodine in the soil. The addition of iodine to salt has prevented goiters in the children.

Pesticides are widely used to control mosquitoes and agricultural pests, but the farmers receive little education on their safe use. Recently, a new road was built, connecting Sharma's village with the neighboring towns. Despite the advantages of having the new road, cars and trucks now speed through her village, rarely stopping to let people cross the road.

In Sharma's village, life expectancy is 49 years. Babies often die of diarrheal diseases in the first year of their lives, and mothers occasionally die from childbirth. Malaria is widespread and hookworm disease is present among those who farm the fields and in children, whose ability to learn is often affected. Malnutrition is also widespread despite the fact that farming is the major occupation in the village.

Chronic lung disease among adults and asthma among the young is surprisingly common, even though cigarette smoking is rare. TB is widespread and is a major cause of death despite the fact that until recently, there have been few cases of HIV/AIDS in the area. Unexplained neurological diseases among farmworkers occur regularly. The most common cause of death among teenagers is motor vehicle injuries along the new road, even though there is only one truck in the village.

Discussion Questions

1. What environmental risk factors contributing to disease and other health conditions are illustrated in this case? Classify each as an unaltered, altered, or built environment factor.
2. Discuss at least two examples of how disease or other conditions found in the village can be explained by the environmental risk factors.
3. Identify at least two interventions that would make a large difference in the health of this village. Classify the interventions as primary, secondary, or tertiary interventions and identify the target group, i.e., individuals, high-risk populations, or general population.

(continues)

$\mathcal{P}$ CASE STUDIES AND DISCUSSION QUESTIONS (continued)

What to Do About Lyme Disease?

You have just moved into a new subdivision—your first home with your young family. The first week you are there, a neighbor tells you that her son has developed Lyme disease and now has chronic arthritis that requires extensive treatment.

Lyme disease is an increasingly common disease that can cause acute and chronic arthritis if not treated early and correctly. In rare instances, it can cause life-threatening heart disease and temporary paralysis often to one side of the face due to nerve damage. The disease is caused by an organism in the spirochete family, which is spread from deer ticks to humans via tick bites. Lyme disease is especially common in communities with large deer populations, which today includes much of the suburban United States as well as rural areas.

Ticks must remain in place on the human skin at least 12–24 hours to extract human blood and inject the spirochete organism at the site of the bite. Complete removal of the small but visible tick within 24 hours usually prevents the disease. Deer ticks are most abundant in the late spring and tend to live on tall grasses from which they can easily move to the bare legs of children and adults.

The disease frequently first appears as a circular red rash around the site of the bite. At this stage, early diagnosis and treatment with antibiotics is usually successful. Several weeks or months later, the onset of arthritis may occur and can be difficult to diagnose. A missed diagnosis may result in severe arthritis that is difficult to treat. A vaccine has been developed and briefly marketed to prevent the disease, but it was quite expensive and only partially successful.

In your new hometown, the local health department is charged with developing a plan for control or elimination of Lyme disease. You are invited to give input on the plan, identifying possible interventions.

Discussion Questions

1. What primary interventions would you consider? Explain.
2. What secondary interventions would you consider? Explain.
3. What tertiary interventions would you consider? Explain.
4. What education, motivation, or obligation approaches do you recommend? Explain.

References

1. University of Wisconsin. Population health sciences. Improving population health. http://www.improvingpopulationhealth.org/blog/what-is-population-health.html. Accessed June 14, 2018.
2. Preamble to the Constitution of WHO as adopted by the International Health Conference, New York, 19 June–22 July 1946; signed on 22 July 1946 by the representatives of 61 States (Official Records of WHO, no. 2, p. 100) and entered into force on 7 April 1948.
3. Public Health Agency of Canada. Population health approach—what determines health? http://www.phac-aspc.gc.ca/ph-sp. Accessed June 14, 2018.

4. Commission on Social Determinants of Health. Closing the gap in a generation: health equity through action on the social determinants of health. *Final Report of the Commission on Social Determinants of Health.* Geneva: World Health Organization; 2008.

5. U.S. Census Bureau. International Database. https://www.census.gov/data-tools/demo/idb/informationGateway.php. Accessed June 14, 2018.

6. Omran AR. The epidemiological transition: a theory of the epidemiology of population change. *Milbank Memorial Fund Q.* 1971;49(4):509–538.

7. Gordis L. *Epidemiology.* 5th ed. Philadelphia, PA: Elsevier Saunders; 2014.

8. Friis RH, Sellers TA. *Epidemiology for Public Health Practice.* 5th ed. Burlington, MA: Jones & Bartlett Learning; 2013.

9. Skolnik R. *Global Health 101.* 3rd ed. Burlington, MA: Jones & Bartlett Learning; 2016.

10. World Health Organization. Healthy life expectancy (HLE) at birth (years). World Health Statistics 2016. http://www.who.int/gho/publications/world_health_statistics/2016/en/. Accessed July 16, 2018.

11. World Health Organization. Global burden of disease. http://www.who.int/topics/global_burden_of_disease/en/. Accessed June 14, 2018.

12. Ramirez, VB. What is R_0?: Gauging contagious infections. Healthline. http://www.healthline.com/health/r-nought-reproduction-number#R0values2. Accessed July 16, 2018.

13. Lamb E. Understand the measles outbreak with this one weird number: the basic reproduction number and why it matters. *Scientific American.* January 31, 2015. http://blogs.scientificamerican.com/roots-of-unity/understand-the-measles-outbreak-with-this-one-weird-number/. Accessed June 14, 2018.

14. Diekmann O, Heesterbeek JAP, Metz JAJ. On the definition and the computation of the basic reproduction ratio R_0 in models for infectious diseases in heterogeneous populations. *J Math Biol.* 1990;28:365–382.

UNIT 2

Systems-Thinking and Systems-Doing

Systems-thinking and systems-doing are key frameworks of population health. Together, they provide the foundation for population health sciences, including the analysis of complex health problems and the identification of potential solutions. As we will see, systems-thinking can be applied to a wide range of health problems, from diseases such as coronary artery disease and HIV/AIDS to social and healthcare issues such as motor vehicle injuries, patient safety, and the excess cost of health care.

Systems-thinking is a way of structuring our thinking about health problems, looking for effective ways to address these problems, and measuring the success of our interventions. Systems-thinking can often help us understand what is needed for successful implementation. We will call this process systems-doing. Therefore, understanding systems-thinking is central to today's population health. Let's start by examining what we mean by a system.

▶ What Is a System?

To understand what we mean by systems-thinking, we need to first discuss what we mean by a system. We will define a **system** as an interacting group of items forming a unified whole.[1] According to O'Connor and McDermott, the key to identifying a system is that a system maintains its existence and functions through the interaction of its parts. They write that the human body is a perfect example of a system:

> Your thoughts affect your digestion and heartbeat, the state of your diges-
> tion affects your thoughts—especially after a large lunch. The eye cannot
> see, nor the legs move without a blood supply, and the blood supply has to
> be oxygenated through the lungs. The movement of the legs helps pump
> the blood back to the heart. The body is a complex system.[2]

It is important to appreciate the features and the implications of a system. O'Connor and McDermott go on to distinguish a system from what they call a heap or collection of pieces, as follows:

- A system is a series of interconnected functioning parts. A heap is merely a collection of parts.
- In a system, the arrangement of the pieces is crucial and the parts work together, while in a heap, the arrangement is irrelevant.
- A system changes if you take away or add pieces; if you cut a system in half, you do not get two smaller systems: you get a system that will not function. A heap can be divided into pieces, each of which can function on its own.
- The behavior of a system depends on its overall structure, while in a heap, size rather than structure determines behavior.

Many structures created by human beings can be thought of as a system. We talk about the educational system, the legal system, as well as the healthcare system and the public health system. Each of these uses of the term "system" shares the goal of understanding how the pieces fit together and interact to produce an outcome.

In population health, we focus on health outcomes. The determinants of health and disease include biological, behavioral, environmental, and social influences. Systems-thinking provides a structured method for organizing these various influences so that we better understand their impacts and assess the potential **effective-ness** of interventions on health outcomes.

▶ What Are the Steps in Systems-Thinking?

Systems-thinking is a structured process that begins by identifying the factors or influences that are believed to lead to an outcome or endpoint. This outcome might be a disease, the outcome of a disease, or a related outcome, such as the cost of health care. The process of systems-thinking goes on to analyze how the factors or influences work together to produce outcomes and how these interactions might change over time. Finally, systems-thinking tries to identify points in the system where interventions might be especially effective in improving outcome. These points are called **bottlenecks** and **leverage points**.

Systems-thinking often proceeds using the following six steps[2,3,*]:

- Step 1: Identify the key factors or influences that impact an outcome such as disease or the outcome of disease.
- Step 2: Indicate the relative strength of the impact of each of the influences or interventions.
- Step 3: Identify how these influences or interventions interact—that is, how they work together.
- Step 4: Identify the dynamic changes that may occur in a system by identifying the feedback loops that occur in the system.
- Step 5: Identify bottlenecks that limit the effectiveness of the system.
- Step 6: Identify leverage points that provide opportunities to greatly improve outcomes.

Let's take a look at each of these steps using cigarette smoking as an example.

Step 1: How Do We Identify Factors or Influences to Include in Systems-Thinking?

Careful selection of the factors or influences to incorporate into systems-thinking is key to the success of the process. It is important to select a limited number of factors that help explain a substantial percent of the outcome. Aiming to explain all outcomes is usually unrealistic and extremely complicated. For instance, when addressing the influences on smoking cessation, we might identify the following interventions as influences that have been shown to have efficacy:

- Smoking cessation programs
- Prohibitions on smoking in public places
- Antitobacco marketing
- Cigarette taxes

While these are not the only factors that affect smoking cessation, the research literature suggests that all of these factors work to reduce cigarette smoking and are realistic interventions to address the problem.

Step 2: How Do We Measure the Strength of the Impacts?

The second step in systems-thinking is to estimate the strength of the relationship between a factor and a disease or between an intervention and an outcome. **Relative risk** is often used to measure the probability of disease or an outcome if an influence is present compared to the probability if the influence is absent. For instance, cigarette smoking of one pack per day for 40 years carries a relative risk of approximately 10. This means that, on average, those who smoke one pack per day for 40 years have

---

* These six steps are often referred to as **systems analysis**. The results of systems analysis may be displayed graphically as systems diagrams. A full systems analysis requires data on the magnitude of each of the factors and their interactions as well as the strength of the feedback loops. Therefore, a complete systems analysis is rarely possible. Nonetheless, systems analysis can help identify bottlenecks and leverage points.

approximately 10 times the probability of developing lung cancer compared to those who never smoked cigarettes. In contrast, the same degree of cigarette smoking carries approximately a relative risk of two for coronary artery disease.[†]

Identifying the influences and the magnitude of the impact is key to systems-thinking, whether we are dealing with a disease, the outcome of a disease, or an outcome such as costs. **BOX 2-1** looks at an example of how systems-thinking has been used to identify the factors or influences and the magnitude of excess costs of the U.S. healthcare system.

In systems-thinking, it is important that we look at the impacts of multiple factors or influences and see how they work together as parts of systems. Therefore, we need to move on to step 3, which looks at the interactions between the influences.

Step 3: How Can We Understand the Interactions between Factors or Influences?

To understand how influences interact, let's take a deeper look at the problem of cigarette smoking. Let's assume that smoking cessation programs, prohibition on smoking in public, anti-tobacco marketing, and higher taxes have been identified as the four most important interventions or influences on the rate of cigarette smoking. The question then becomes how they can be effectively and efficiently combined.

We might start by adding together the impact of each influence or intervention. That is, we could assume what is called a **straight-line relationship** or linear relationship between influences. A straight-line relationship implies that increased levels of an intervention, such as increasing taxes on tobacco, will produce a straight-line decrease in the levels of tobacco use. However, it is possible that small increases in taxes have little effect, while somewhat larger increases have dramatic effects.

Thus, systems-thinking asks questions about how to most effectively utilize cigarette taxes by varying the amount of the tax and by combining taxes with other approaches, such as using the taxes to support tobacco education programs.

Looking at the interactions between diseases is especially important when the impact of two conditions or diseases multiples the risk. This is the situation with cigarettes and radon and also with cigarettes and asbestos. Say, the relative risk for cigarette smoking is 10 for lung cancer, and the relative risk for either radon exposure or asbestos for lung cancer is 5. If cigarette smoking plus one of the other conditions is present, the relative risk is approximately 50. Reduction or elimination of any of these risk factors can have a dramatic impact on the incidence of lung cancer because of these **multiplicative interactions**.

---

† Relative risk may also be presented as a number between 0 and 1. This occurs when the factor that increases risk is in the denominator. This may occur when a factor reduces the risk, such as exercise and coronary artery disease, or when an intervention results in reduced risk. **Odds ratios** may be used as a good approximation of relative risk except when the probability of disease is very high. An increased relative risk does not in-and-of-itself imply the presence of a cause and effect relationship.

BOX 2-1 Factors Producing Excess Costs of Health Care in the United States

The Institute of Medicine, now known as the National Academy of Medicine, took a systems-thinking approach to identifying the factors that influence the excess costs of the U.S. healthcare system.[4] Excess costs can be thought of as expenditures that do not improve population health. For each category or factor, they identified the types of excess costs that occur. In addition, they estimated the magnitude of the estimated potential annual savings from each of the six categories of excess costs.

Unnecessary services and overuse—beyond evidence-established levels—$210 billion

- Discretionary use beyond benchmarks
- Unnecessary choice of higher-cost services

Inefficiently delivered services—$130 billion

- Mistakes—errors, preventable complications
- Care fragmentation
- Unnecessary use of higher-cost providers
- Operational inefficiencies at care delivery sites

Excess administrative costs—$190 billion

- Insurance paperwork costs
- Insurers' administrative inefficiencies
- Inefficiencies due to care documentation requirements

Prices that are too high—$105 billion

- Service prices beyond competitive benchmarks
- Product prices beyond competitive benchmarks

Missed prevention opportunities—$55 billion

- Primary prevention
- Secondary prevention
- Tertiary prevention

Fraud—$75 billion

- All sources—payers, clinicians, patients

Together, these excess costs come to approximately 25% of the dollars the United States spends on health care. Systems-thinking efforts to reduce these costs provide great opportunities for controlling healthcare costs without jeopardizing quality or access.*

Data from Institute of Medicine. The Healthcare Imperative: Lowering Costs and Improving Outcomes-Workshop Series Summary. Available at: https://www.nap.edu/catalog/12750/the-healthcare-imperative-lowering-costs-and-improving-outcomes-workshop-series. Accessed July 16, 2018.

---

* These figures reflect 2009 expenditures and therefore underestimate today's potential dollar saving, though the conclusion that approximately 25% of the dollars the United States spends on health care can be considered excess costs is likely to still be accurate.

Step 4: How Do We Identify the Dynamic Changes That Occur in a System?

Systems-thinking requires not only an examination of multiple influences and their interactions at one point in time using a static approach, but also encourages us to look at how these factors change over time. That is, systems-thinking takes a dynamic approach.

Systems-thinking attempts to take into account changes in the overall system that occur over time due to changes in one or more of the factors or influences. These changes in a factor or influence are often the result of changes in one factor due to changes in another factor. This process is known as feedback, and it produces what are called **feedback loops**.

In biological systems, a feedback loop may occur, for example, when there is blood loss, and vasoconstriction occurs to at least temporarily counter the blood loss. Another feedback loop occurs in response to high atmospheric temperatures. In hot environments, the body increases sweating, concentrates urine, conserves energy, and hopefully gets out of the sun, which together may effectively reduce the physiological impact of heat.

Feedback loops also exist when we are talking about health problems such as the impact of cigarettes. We might ask: does the reduction in the percentage of people who smoke due to higher taxes lead to changes over time in social attitudes, which themselves may set the stage for greater enforcement of public smoking regulations? This type of feedback is known as a positive feedback loop because the initial change leads to another change in the same direction.

Alternatively, raising cigarette taxes might reduce the money available to low-income individuals to pay for smoking cessation programs, especially if these services are not paid for by health insurance. This type of feedback is known as a negative feedback loop because the initial change leads to another change in the opposite direction.

Similarly, communicable disease in a population is controlled to a certain extent by responses or feedback, including voluntary isolation of sick individuals, development of immunity, and unfortunately, death of affected individuals. Understanding these feedback loops can help us improve on the natural systems that exist, while building on the positive aspects of existing systems, such as the development of immunity.

Systems-thinking does more than look at how a system operates at one point in time. Identifying feedback loops is key to understanding how a system operates and changes over time. Understanding feedback and the changes it can produce is a prerequisite for the next steps in systems-thinking, predicting how a system changes over time.

Steps 5 and 6: What Are Bottlenecks and Leverage Points?

Looking at the feedback loops and the changes that occur over time allows us to identify bottlenecks. Bottlenecks are points in a system, such as the narrowing in an hour glass or a traffic jam, which limits the speed or effectiveness of a system. Removal of a bottleneck may greatly speed up the system and improve the outcome of a system.

For instance, systems-thinking might identify a bottleneck such as the need to train large numbers of clinicians in smoking cessation methods so that they can address the demand for smoking cessation services created by anti-tobacco marketing, increased cigarette taxes, and better drug treatments.

A leverage point is a point in the system where a large improvement in outcome can be obtained from a modest improvement in a factor. For instance, with cigarette smoking, we might identify smoking during pregnancy as a leverage point. Pregnant women who smoke are often highly motivated to quit due to the severe impact on their offspring. The impact of modest investment in smoking cessation efforts for pregnant women may have large short-term impacts on a newborn as well as long-term impacts on the mother.

Now we have identified the six steps in systems-thinking. Let's use these six steps of systems-thinking to help us apply systems-thinking to coronary artery disease.

▶ How Can We Apply the Six Systems-Thinking Steps to the Problem of Coronary Artery Disease?

We might apply systems-thinking to the problem of coronary artery disease using the six steps, as follows:

Step 1: Identify influences—There are multiple factors that increase the risk of coronary artery disease, including high blood pressure, high low-density lipoprotein (LDL) cholesterol, low high-density lipoprotein (HDL) cholesterol, elevated triglycerides, abdominal obesity, diabetes, cigarette smoking, physical inactivity, and family history.

Step 2: Estimate the relative strength of the influences—We need to estimate the relative strength or magnitude of the impact of each of the influences. We might estimate the relative risk for each of these factors, or we might classify their impacts as weak, moderate, or strong. In the case of coronary artery disease, each of these factors is generally considered of moderate strength with relative risks in the range of 2–4.

Step 3: Examine the interactions between factors—Examining the interaction between factors helps us understand what happens when two or more of the factors are present. Risk factors for disease may add together to increase the risk of disease, or in some cases, they may multiply the risk rather than resulting in an additive impact. Alternatively, one factor, such as physical activity, may have a protective effect against coronary artery disease in and of itself.

Risk factors for coronary artery disease have typically been assumed to add together rather than to multiply the impact. However, a combination of risk factors, known as the metabolic syndrome, has been known to interact and greatly increase the risk. Metabolic syndrome includes increased abdominal obesity, low HDL cholesterol, elevated triglycerides, hypertension, and elevated fasting blood sugar. When all or a number of these risk factors occur together, they increase the probability of an adverse outcome such as coronary artery disease by a greater extent than would be expected by simply adding together the impacts of each of these factors.

Step 4: Identify feedback loops that lead to dynamic changes in the functioning of the system—Understanding how systems operate over time requires us to identify feedback mechanisms, or feedback loops, that alter the likelihood of disease or impact its outcome. For instance, increased weight, especially increased abdominal girth, leads to increased LDL cholesterol, diabetes, reduced exercise, reduced HDL cholesterol, and increased blood pressure. Alternatively, multiple interventions focused on weight, exercise, blood sugar control, and treatment of hypertension may work together to greatly reduce the probability of coronary artery disease.

Step 5: Identify bottlenecks—Bottlenecks imply that there are points in the system that need to be addressed in order for the other factors or influences to have their potential impacts. For instance, in coronary artery disease, if severe narrowing of the coronary arteries already exists, it is unlikely that interventions such as reducing blood sugar, reducing LDL cholesterol, increasing exercise, or stopping cigarette smoking are going to have a dramatic impact. If the bottleneck, the narrowed artery, can be addressed using angioplasty or surgery, attention to the other risk factors may have a much greater impact.

Step 6: Identify leverage points—The systems-thinking that we have done so far suggests some leverage points where interventions may have greater than expected impacts. For instance, increasing exercise post angioplasty or surgery may be safer than when a severe disease is present. Patients may also be highly motivated to exercise after having angioplasty or surgery. Exercise might be effective in helping patients stop smoking cigarettes and reducing abdominal girth as well as having an impact on HDL cholesterol and blood sugar.

Systems-thinking provides a useful method for addressing a wide range of complex health problems. The use of simultaneous interventions and focusing on bottlenecks and leverage points have become highly successful approaches for addressing population health issues. When examining any systems-thinking approach, looking for how bottlenecks and leverage points are identified and addressed is central to understanding the thinking process.

Let's look at additional examples of a range of uses of systems-thinking.

▶ How Can Systems-Thinking Help Us Develop Strategies for Multiple Simultaneous Interventions?

As we have seen, the approach to coronary artery disease has successfully utilized multiple simultaneous interventions for several decades. Today, we are moving to a coordinated strategy of utilizing interventions throughout the course of disease that can be categorized as primary, secondary, and tertiary interventions. Primary interventions include control of high blood pressure, cholesterol, cigarette smoking, obesity, diabetes, and a growing list of other contributory causes of coronary artery disease.

Secondary interventions designed to prevent heart damage and death—including interventions in the early hours of a myocardial infarction—have become an increasingly successful part of an overall strategy. Drug treatment and postmyocardial exercise rehabilitation are now a standard part of medical care. Finally, tertiary interventions to prevent sudden death in public places have now become a population health intervention, with placement of automated defibrillators in places where people congregate, such as airports and sporting events.

New approaches to disease often combine primary, secondary, and tertiary interventions. For instance, efforts to address HIV may in the future include primary prevention through barrier protection, male circumcision, precoital and intracoital treatment, and eventually vaccination. Postexposure treatments are being extensively investigated as well. Detection during the first few weeks, when transmissibility is greatest, is being investigated as an important new intervention. In addition, early and continuous drug treatment of HIV has been found not only to help the individual, but also to reduce his or her infectivity.

Maternal to child transmission has been viewed as a leverage point in HIV control since it is feasible and affects both the mother and the child. The dramatic reduction in maternal to child transmission of HIV is an example of the potential for multiple interventions to improve outcome. HIV can be transmitted across the placenta during pregnancy. The higher the level of virus in the mother's blood, the greater the probability of transmission. Thus, early testing and active treatment of pregnant women is fundamental to prevention of maternal–child transmission. In addition, there is an increased risk during vaginal delivery. Selective use of cesarean delivery can reduce this risk. Early treatment of infants has been shown to reduce the risk even further. Finally, breastfeeding carries a small but important risk of transmission. Avoidance of breastfeeding or active maternal drug treatment during breastfeeding among women with HIV can greatly reduce this risk as well. Today, HIV infection by the maternal–child route should be considered a failure of population health.

The strategy of coordinated use of multiple simultaneous complementary interventions has become a highly successful population health strategy. For many years, interventions were studied and applied one intervention at a time, with little thought about how they interact or how they could be used in combination to produce the best results. In recent years, systems-thinking approaches have contributed to the development of increasingly effective strategies that combine multiple interventions.

▶ How Can Systems-Thinking Help Identify Bottlenecks and Leverage Points That Can Be Used to Improve Population Health?

Identifying bottleneck and leverage points can be extremely helpful in guiding the development of interventions. Motor vehicle injuries provide an important example of the key role played by bottlenecks and leverage points.

In the 1960s, it was recognized that after trauma, such as injuries from war or motor vehicle collisions, many victims are able to physiologically respond and temporarily tolerate blood loss and other injuries before rapidly deteriorating. This early period became known as the "golden hour."

Few victims of motor vehicle injuries before the 1970s were reaching emergency care during the golden hour. To address this bottleneck, a sophisticated system of emergency response was put into place in the United States, which greatly reduced the response time and resulted in a large-scale reduction in deaths and disabilities from motor vehicle collisions.

In contrast, leverage points are points in systems in which successful interventions produce better than expected outcomes. We can see them as opportunities to make major improvements in outcomes. At leverage points, there is no bottleneck, but the conditions are right to take advantage of the interactions that exist between factors.

For instance, a leverage point for reduced motor vehicle injuries has been the impact of alcohol. Alcohol consumption affects speed and response time and, in the not-too-distant past, was a contributory cause of a large percentage of deaths and disabilities due to motor vehicle collisions. The combination of legal enforcement, consumption of lower alcohol content beverages, and cultural changes, such as the use of designated drivers, has had a dramatic impact on mortality from motor vehicle injuries.

In addition to the successful application of systems-thinking to multiple intervention strategies and the focus on bottlenecks and leverage points, systems-thinking has been important in understanding and addressing the spread of disease.

▶ How Can Systems-Thinking Be Used to Address the Spread of Disease?

Communicable diseases are inherently population health issues since they may produce the spread of disease in a population. Systems-thinking has been an underpinning of our approach to communicable disease as a population health problem.

It is well known that the occurrence of immunity by vaccination, disease exposure, and other mechanisms prevents the incidence of disease from continuing to increase. This process, known as **herd immunity**, or perhaps better called population immunity, is the basis for many vaccine-based population health interventions, including measles, mumps, chickenpox, and other vaccine preventable diseases with a large R naught. Population immunity implies that if a high enough percentage of the population has effective immunity, the spread of disease in that population will be suppressed and an epidemic will be prevented. Thus, providing widespread vaccination can address a bottleneck for control of many vaccine preventable diseases.

In recent years, it has become clear that some of our most difficult noncommunicable disease problems can also spread in populations. Population health is beginning to extend the concept of population immunity to noncommunicable diseases. Obesity and the opioid crisis are good examples of noncommunicable disease problems that need to be addressed using a systems-thinking and population perspective as well as an individual perspective.

There is increasingly strong evidence that conditions such as obesity and opioid overdoses are greatly affected by relationships or networks of individuals. While this has probably always been true to some extent, today's instantaneous communications and social networks are rapidly expanding the interpersonal influences of high-risk behaviors. This process is called **interference**, and it may explain unexpected or exponential increases in conditions or diseases. It may also provide new methods for intervening to interrupt the spread of noncommunicable diseases.

Finally, systems-thinking may help us move from looking at one problem at a time to developing an approach for the overall workings of a system.

▶ How Can Systems-Thinking Help Us Improve the Overall Workings of Systems?

Systems-thinking approaches to food safety have been increasingly successful in recent years in reducing the rates of hospitalization and death from foodborne illness. These approaches identified bottlenecks and leverage points for special attention. Initially, systems-thinking focused on identifying interventions for high-risk foods one type of food at a time. Later, it went on to take a fully developed systems-thinking approach to food safety. This process has been called the Hazard Analysis and Critical Control Points (HACCP) system.[5]

HACCP is a systems-thinking approach that looks for bottlenecks and leverage points to manage food safety issues. It starts by removing bottlenecks to food safety by first ensuring basic environmental and operating conditions. These include facilities that maintain sanitary conditions; proper equipment construction, installation, and maintenance; and personal hygiene by employees. Once these basic conditions of food safety are accomplished, HACCP looks for options for interventions at multiple leverage or control points and institutes a series of safeguards at these specific points.

Meat safety issues reflect this approach. Ground beef, which often combines meat from leftover portions of multiple animals, has been identified as a high-risk product or hazard. The reduction in risk has been viewed as a leverage point. Toxin-producing strains of *Escherichia coli* were previously widespread in ground beef products and have been responsible for a number of fatal outbreaks of foodborne illness in the past. The threats to health have led to a more coordinated systems-thinking approach using the HACCP system.

Key leverage points at which ground beef may be contaminated in the meat-packing process have been identified for special emphasis. Monitoring by testing now includes a random testing process on all batches of ground beef. The process uses rapid testing of a sample of the finished ground beef and holding up distribution until the results are available. Education of consumers about the danger of eating rare or raw ground beef is also a key leverage point in this strategy. In addition, separating beef products from other food preparation, especially from food products eaten raw, is an important educational effort.

HACCP is increasingly being adopted for products such as seafood, meat, poultry, and fruit juices. The HACCP process has already had a major impact on the incidence of disease associated with ground beef. It is not a cure-all, but looking at the process has helped us come up with effective interventions.

New approaches to food safety build on the HACCP system and its big-picture look at the entire process. In the past, identifying the source of food contamination has been a bottleneck in investigation of foodborne outbreaks. In an emerging systems-thinking approach, most food's detailed location and time of production down to the level of the farm or factory are being identified on the label. This allows public health officials to trace the food back to where and when the problem occurred.

Adding this approach to the HACCP provides a mechanism for quickly responding to early indications of foodborne outbreaks, regardless of the type of food involved. The combination of the HACCP system and food tracing provides the potential for a fully developed systems-thinking approach to food safety.

Another example of the application of systems-thinking to improving the operations of an overall system is the patient safety movement, which seeks to improve the outcomes of the healthcare system by taking a systems-thinking approach. **BOX 2-2** provides an overview of this important advance in the delivery of health care.

Finally, a systems-thinking approach called **One Health** has recently been developed to address the increasingly important issues related to the biggest system of all: the system that includes humans, animals, and the ecosystem.

BOX 2-2 Patient Safety Movement

The patient safety movement began in the early years of the 21st century with the report of the National Academy of Medicine titled *To Err is Human: Building a Safer Health System*.[6] The report found that approximately 100,000 deaths per year in hospitals alone are the result of errors. Medication errors, equipment malfunctions, and interprofessional communication or "handoff errors" are among the most common errors leading to preventable adverse events. More recently, an emphasis on diagnostic errors has become a focus as well.

The patient safety movement has shifted the focus from errors to safety. That is, it is built on the contention that most adverse events are due to **system errors** and are not a personal failure, as the National Academy of Medicine wrote: "the biggest challenge to moving toward a safer health system is changing the culture from one of blaming individuals for errors to one in which errors are treated not as personal failures, but as opportunities to improve the system and prevent harm."[7] Reframing the issue from personal failure to system errors can be viewed as addressing a key bottleneck.

To remove this bottleneck, the patient safety movement has developed what they call a "culture of safety." A culture of safety is built on the three principles taken from the National Academy of Medicine report: trust, accountability, and transparency. A recent patient safety movement summary of a culture of safety calls for the following actions[8]:

- Achieving a culture of safety in a healthcare organization requires transformational change that is owned and led by the top leaders of the organization, including the board. Leaders cannot simply be "on board" with patient safety—they must own it.
- Transparency, both within and outside of the organization, drives improvement across the continuum of care.
- If patient harm results from a medical error, apologize in 30 minutes, pay for all care, seek a just resolution, provide a credit card for future care of the survivor of harm.
- Creating reliable means to capture and analyze good catches/near misses is the key to identifying and addressing unstable processes and systems.
- Both safety culture and patient outcomes require continual assessment: "What is measured gets managed."

The patient safety movement has benefited from the experience of complex nonmedical industries, such as the airline industry, which have evolved incident reporting systems that can be viewed as leverage points for safety since they do the following[9]:

- Focus on the large number of near misses
- Provide incentives for voluntary reporting

- Ensure confidentiality while bolstering accountability
- Emphasize perspectives of systems in data collection, analysis, and improvement

Attention to near misses provides greater frequency of events allowing quantitative analysis; limits legal liability; and allows investigation of recovery patterns that can be captured, studied, and used for improvement. The shift to reporting and investigating near misses has been a leverage point for improving patient safety as well as airline safety.

The patient safety movement is now a full-fledged part of the healthcare system. It is beginning to have important impacts on the number of adverse events, the costs of health care, and the role of the malpractice system.

▶ How Can Systems-Thinking Help Us Understand the Relationship Between Human Health, Animal Health, and Ecosystem Health?

The One Health movement is a population health movement that uses systems-thinking to understand the impacts of the connections between human, animal, and ecosystem health, as illustrated in **FIGURE 2-1**.

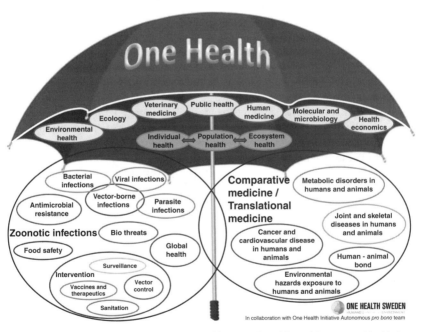

FIGURE 2-1 Relationships between Human Health, Animal Health, and Ecosystem Health Are Central to One Health

Reproduced from One Health Sweden. Http://www.onehealthinitiative.com/about.php

One Health is about the larger system: the world we live in. The One Health movement asserts that human health is dependent on animal health as well as the health of the ecosystem.

It has been a response to increasing threats of emerging and reemerging infectious diseases, from AIDS and SARS to Ebola and Zika, which have spilled over from animals and the ecosystem to become important human diseases. Antibiotic resistance, climate change, globalization, and other disruptions in animals and the ecosystem likewise pose increasing risks to human health.[10]

One Health looks primarily at the following three components:

- Microbiological influences on health and disease
- Ecosystem health
- Human–animal interaction

Let's take a brief look at each of the components of One Health.[‡]

▶ What Are the Most Important Microbiological Threats to Human Health?

A wide range of microbiological entities can produce human disease, including DNA and RNA viruses, bacteria, a wide range of parasites, protozoa, and fungi, as well as prions, which are a disease-causing form of a normal brain protein.

Many of the most serious microbiological threats to the population's health are due to RNA viruses. An **RNA virus** is far more likely than a DNA virus to produce mutations during the frequent replications since it does not have the same protective mechanism against copying or coding errors. This high rate of mutation in RNA viruses is believed to enhance their ability to cross species lines and to continue to mutate once established in a new species. There are currently approximately 200 species of RNA viruses that can infect humans, and more species are being added each year. This represents only a small fraction of the RNA viruses that exist in nature.[11]

RNA viruses, however, account for most of the emerging infectious diseases that have spilled over from animals to humans in recent years.[12] Therefore, putting a focus on RNA viruses can be viewed as a leverage point in a systems-thinking approach. These include the following:

- AIDS/human immunodeficiency virus (HIV)
- Chikungunya
- Ebola
- Middle Eastern respiratory syndrome (MERS)
- Severe acute respiratory syndrome (SARS)

---

‡ One Health has been defined as "the collaborative effort of multiple health science professions, together with their related disciplines and institutions to obtain optimal health for people, domestic animals, wildlife, plants, and our environment."[10] We will examine the One Health movement from the perspective of human health. However, ideally, these benefits flow both ways. Animals may benefit from control of zoonotic diseases and from the human–animal bond. In addition, reducing the rate of human-mediated species loss and artificial introduction of nonnative species may help sustain ecosystems.

- West Nile virus
- Zika virus

In addition, Influenza A, with its ability to infect animals and mutate to allow person-to-person spread, represents an ongoing threat to human health.

▶ What Is the Impact of Ecosystem Health on Human Health?

Ecosystem health and its impact on human health involves a wide range of factors that directly affect the physical world in which we live. These impacts stem from the following factors[12,13]:

- *Global movement of populations*: Major migrations of human populations and exposures to new disease have been a major population health issue since the European diseases of tuberculosis (TB) and smallpox killed tens of millions of Native Americans in North and South America. The increasing speed and numbers of people moving across the globe pose new and continuing risks in the 21st century.
- *Agriculture and changes in food distribution*: The U.S. food supply now comes from over 100 countries posing new risks of disease outbreaks ranging from pesticides, food contamination, antibiotic overuse, and an increased risk of Influenza A and other diseases due to concentration of livestock and poultry in feedlots.
- *Ecological changes in land and resource use*: Human interventions in the ecosystem can increase or decrease disease, ranging from the spread of Lyme disease due to deer ticks and the increase in schistosomiasis after construction of dams to reduced infection from Chagas disease with modern home construction methods.
- *Climate change*: Health risks from climate change include the acute impacts of extreme heat, flooding, and pollution from forest fires as well as the chronic impacts on asthma, vectorborne and waterborne diseases and the potential mental health impacts of climate change, such as the stress associated with exposure to extreme weather and disasters.

▶ How Do Human–Animal Interactions Affect Human Health?

The final component of the **One Health Educational Framework** is human–animal interaction. Pet ownership is by far the most common way that most human beings come in contact with animals. Today, nearly two-thirds of Americans own at least one pet.

The National Institutes of Health indicates, "The general belief is that there are health benefits to owning pets, both in terms of psychological growth and development, as well as physical health benefits."[14] Evidence suggests additional benefits, including reduced allergies and asthma among children exposed to pets during the first year of life and increased ability to communicate among children with autism.

While domesticated animals, such as dogs and cats, can provide considerable benefits to humans, they are not free of risk of disease to humans. Dogs, and to a lesser extent cats, are a potential source of rabies. Fortunately, proper vaccinations effectively protect dogs and cats as well as humans. Today, the transmission of rabies to humans from dogs and cats is very rare. The Centers for Disease Control and Prevention (CDC) recognizes a number of other preventable risks, as discussed in **BOX 2-3**.

The preventable diseases caused by cats and dogs are viewed by most Americans as far less of a threat than the many benefits of the human–animal bond. The same cannot be said of other types of pets that the CDC has called "exotic pets."[§]

There are approximately 10 million animals imported into the United States each year, including amphibians, birds, mammals, and reptiles. The risks posed by

---

BOX 2-3 Preventable Human Health Risks from Dogs and Cats

CDC stresses the importance of preventing the following human health risks from dogs and cats:

- Toxoplasmosis is an infection caused by a microscopic parasite called *Toxoplasma gondii*. Toxoplasmosis can cause severe illness in infants, including vision loss and seizures, when infected from their mothers before birth. The most common way for a pregnant woman to become infected is through contact with a cat's litter box. According to the CDC, pregnant women should ideally avoid changing a cat's litter box and avoid adopting stray cats. Everyone should cover outdoor sandboxes to keep cats away.[15]
- Cat-scratch disease (CSD) is a bacterial infection spread by cats. The disease spreads when an infected cat licks a person's open wound or bites or scratches a person hard enough to break the surface of the skin, often leading to spread of the infection to the lymph nodes. Washing cat bites and scratches well with soap and running water helps prevent human disease. People should not allow cats to lick human wounds. About 40% of cats carry the disease-producing bacteria *B. henselae* at some time in their lives, although most cats with this infection show no signs of illness.[16]
- Toxocariasis is a preventable parasitic infection caused by the larval form of the dog or cat roundworms *Toxocara canis* and *Toxocara cati*. *Toxocara* eggs are often found in dog feces and, occasionally, cat feces. People can acquire toxocariasis if they accidentally come in skin contact with or ingest dirt containing *Toxocara* eggs after gardening or playing in dirt or sand contaminated with infected feces. After skin contact with the *Toxocara* eggs, the larvae hatch and may travel under the skin (cutaneous larva migrans or creeping eruption). Toxocariasis can rarely invade the eyes and other organs, including the brain, where severe damage can occur. Preventive measures greatly reduce the risk of toxocariasis. These measures include controlling *Toxocara* infection in dogs and cats through deworming by a veterinarian and reducing contact with the larvae by promptly disposing of dog and cat feces to a place away from people.[17]

---

§ The term "exotic pet" has no single definition; it can refer to any native or nonnative wildlife kept in human households, including domestic reptiles and amphibians. Small domestic mammals may or may not be classified as exotic pets.

this type of exotic pet ownership illustrates the components of One Health, including risks to humans, animals, and the ecosystem. For example, monkeypox, a less severe relative of smallpox, has been spread by imported pets. Pet pythons that have been released into wetlands have become unchecked predators. Lionfish, an invasive marine species common in the aquarium trade, are now threatening reefs throughout the Caribbean and Gulf of Mexico due to release by pet owners in Florida. A focus on exotic pets represents a leverage point in a systems-thinking approach.

The One Health movement may be seen as the ultimate effort to view the health of the public as part of one large system in which we all live. The One Health movement provides an opportunity to look at the interactions between human health, animal health, and ecosystem health and identify bottlenecks and leverage points. The One Health movement is helping us understand that addressing microbiological threats, the impact of ecosystem change, and the impacts of close human-animal interactions is key to developing a healthy planet. We are "all in it together" is no longer just about the human race; it is about the health of all living things.

Our look at systems-thinking should make it clear that we need to connect the components of the health system and connect the health system with the broader society and world we live in. Systems-thinking provides the structure for considering options for implementation to address population health problems. An important and often missing component of implementation is coordination across the pillars of population health, i.e., health care, public health, and health policy. Therefore, in addressing implementation based on systems-thinking, we will focus on the possible methods for interprofessional coordination. We will call this coordination **systems-doing**.

▶ What Do We Mean by Systems-Doing and How Can We Use It to Connect the Components of the Health System?

The days when the right hand of the health system does not know what the left hand is doing need to come to an end. Computer technology, including electronic health records, can help make this happen, but interprofessional collaboration and organizational restructuring, such as the development of integrated healthcare systems, are also needed before systems-thinking can maximize its impact on improving population health.

Understanding health systems using systems-thinking goes a long way in helping us think of options for intervention. Thinking of options, however, is not an end in itself. Effectively implementing interventions requires more than systems-thinking; it requires what we will call systems-doing. Systems-doing often requires a coordinated effort between professions to more successfully connect components of a larger system.

The healthcare and public health systems have long been two separate systems, with the healthcare system often consuming over 95% of the dollars spent on health. Systems-thinking challenges us to see the healthcare system and the public health system as two components of the larger health system. Systems-doing requires us to understand these systems, understand their connections, and focus on what needs to be done to make them work together more effectively and efficiently.

Connecting the components of a system starts with an understanding of what each component of the system does. Clinicians and healthcare administrators are often not fully aware of the role played by the public health system and vice versa. **Essential Health Benefits** and **Essential Public Health Services** are useful summaries of the roles played by the healthcare and public health systems as part of population health.⸕

BOX 2-4 outlines the Essential Health Benefits that have come to define the scope of healthcare services needed by the population as a whole.

The public health system also has its list of 10 essentials. These are services provided primarily to groups or populations rather than specific individuals. **TABLE 2-1** outlines the 10 Essential Public Health Services and provides a definition and examples of each essential service.[19]

BOX 2-4 Essential Health Benefits

Essential Health Benefits are defined as healthcare services provided to individuals. They include each of the following 10 categories of health services[18]:

1. Ambulatory patient services (outpatient services)
2. Emergency services
3. Hospitalization
4. Maternity and newborn care
5. Mental health and substance use disorder services, including behavioral health treatment
6. Prescription drugs
7. Rehabilitative and habilitative services (those that help patients acquire, maintain, or improve skills necessary for daily functioning) and devices
8. Laboratory services
9. Preventive and wellness services and chronic disease management
10. Pediatric services, including oral and vision care

This list of services was developed as part of the Affordable Care Act and is an example of criteria against which comprehensive health care and comprehensive health insurance can be judged. It aims to cover the services that should be included in comprehensive health care, whether or not a particular individual may potentially need the service. For instance, insurance for older women includes pregnancy services and insurance for healthy individuals includes habilitative and rehabilitative services so that everyone shares the costs and reduces the overall cost of insurance.

Additional services ranging from adult oral and vision services, to cosmetic surgery, to experimental treatments may not be covered by the Essential Health Benefits. Importantly, this set of Essential Health Benefits does not include transportation, translation services, and other services that may be required to effectively obtain health care. Nonetheless, defining and incorporating the Essential Health Benefits into health insurance and health care has helped standardize and expand the range of services that are now defined as essential.

⸕ It should be recognized that the Essential Health Benefits and the Essential Public Health services are not completely parallel frameworks. Essential Health Benefits address the outputs of the healthcare system, while the Essential Public Health Services address the services to be provided. Nonetheless, these are useful summaries of what health care and public health see as their essential contributions to population health.

TABLE 2-1 The 10 Essential Public Health Services

Essential service	Meaning of essential service	Examples
Monitor health status to identify and solve community health problems	This service includes accurate diagnosis of the community's health status; identification of threats to health and assessment of health service needs; timely collection, analysis, and publication of information on access, utilization, costs, and outcomes of personal health services; attention to the vital statistics and health status of specific groups that are at a higher risk than the total population; and collaboration to manage integrated information systems with private providers and health benefit plans.	Vital statistics; health surveys; surveillance, including reportable diseases
Diagnose and investigate health problems and health hazards in the community	This service includes epidemiologic identification of emerging health threats; public health laboratory capability using modern technology to conduct rapid screening and high-volume testing; active communicable disease epidemiology programs; and technical capacity for epidemiologic investigation of disease outbreaks and patterns of chronic disease and injury.	Epidemic investigations; CDC–Epidemic Intelligence Service; state public health laboratories
Inform, educate, and empower people about health issues	This service includes social marketing and media communications; providing accessible health information resources at community levels; active collaboration with personal healthcare providers to reinforce health promotion messages and programs; and joint health education programs with schools, churches, and worksites.	Health education campaigns, such as comprehensive state tobacco programs

(continues)

TABLE 2-1 The 10 Essential Public Health Services   *(continued)*

Essential service	Meaning of essential service	Examples
Mobilize community partnerships and action to identify and solve health problems	This service includes convening and facilitating community groups and associations, including those not typically considered to be health-related, in undertaking defined preventive, screening, rehabilitation, and support programs; and skilled coalition-building to draw upon the full range of potential human and material resources in the cause of community health.	Lead control programs: testing and follow-up of children, reduction of lead exposure, educational follow-up, and addressing underlying causes
Develop policies and plans that support individual and community health efforts	This service requires leadership development at all levels of public health; systematic community and state-level planning for health improvement in all jurisdictions; tracking of measurable health objectives as a part of continuous quality improvement strategies; joint evaluation with the medical/healthcare system to define consistent policy regarding prevention and treatment services; and development of codes, regulations, and legislation to guide public health practice.	Newborn screening and follow-up programs for phenylketonuria (PKU) and other genetic and congenital diseases
Enforce laws and regulations that protect health and ensure safety	This service involves full enforcement of sanitary codes, especially in the food industry; full protection of drinking water supplies; enforcement of clean air standards; timely follow-up of hazards, preventable injuries, and exposure-related diseases identified in occupational and community settings; monitoring quality of medical services (e.g., laboratory, nursing home, and home health care); and timely review of new drug, biological, and medical device applications.	Local: Fluoridation and chlorination of water; state: Regulation of nursing homes; federal: FDA drug approval and food safety

Link people to needed personal health services and ensure the provision of health care when otherwise unavailable	This service (often referred to as "outreach" or "enabling" services) includes ensuring effective entry for socially disadvantaged people into a coordinated system of clinical care; culturally and linguistically appropriate materials and staff to ensure linkage to services for special population groups; ongoing "care management"; and transportation.	Community health centers
Ensure the provision of a competent public and personal healthcare workforce	This service includes education and training for personnel to meet the needs of public and personal health services; efficient processes for licensure of professionals and certification of facilities with regular verification and inspection follow-up; adoption of continuous quality improvement and lifelong learning within all licensure and certification programs; active partnerships with professional training programs to ensure community-relevant learning experiences for all students; and continuing education in management and leadership development programs for those charged with administrative/executive roles.	Licensure of physicians, nurses, and other health professionals
Evaluate effectiveness, accessibility, and quality of personal and population-based health services	This service calls for ongoing evaluation of health programs, based on analysis of health status and service utilization data, to assess program effectiveness and provide information necessary for allocating resources and reshaping programs.	Development of evidence-based recommendations
Research for new insights and innovative solutions to health problems	This service includes continuous linkage with appropriate institutions of higher learning and research and an internal capacity to mount timely epidemiologic and economic analyses and conduct required health services research.	NIH, CDC, AHRQ, other federal agencies

Data from the Public Health System and the 10 Essential Public Health Services. Available at https://www.cdc.gov/stltpublichealth/publichealthservices/essentialhealthservices.html. Accessed June 15, 2018.

▶ # What Strategies Can We Use to Connect the Components of the Health System?

Now that we've seen the different services provided by the healthcare system and the public health system, let's look at strategies to connect the components. Connecting the components of the health system requires more than understanding the roles played by each of the components. It requires strategies for connecting the components. Let's examine the following three basic systems-doing strategies for coordinating the components of the health system:

- **Parallel play**
- **Collaboration**
- **Integration of efforts**

We will take a look at what we mean by each of the strategies and examine examples of each. In addition, case studies at the end of this unit provide extended examples of systems-doing.

Parallel Play

Parallel play, as the name implies, reflects simultaneous action with little direct connection. With parallel play, the relationships between the components of the system are often minimal, but they are each playing their part in making the overall system function. Ideally, the components are working to achieve the same goals, and their efforts do not interfere with each other.

At times, parallel play is all that is needed and can be quite effective. For many years, this was the relationship between the U.S. healthcare system and the U.S. public health system. At its best, the two systems each went their own way, developed their own organizational structures and education systems, and were each funded through their own funding mechanisms. At times, this parallel play worked reasonably well when efforts were made to develop common goals and avoid potential conflicts.

Examples of successful parallel play include the following.

Coronary Artery Disease

A dramatic reduction in coronary artery disease has occurred over the last 75 years, reducing the mortality rate from coronary artery disease by approximately half. In the 1950s, coronary artery disease caused almost half of all deaths. This especially affected men, who often died suddenly in their 50s and early 60s. Medical interventions, such as coronary care units, by-pass surgery, and angioplasty, have saved and prolonged many lives.

Prevention and public health efforts also play a key role. Reductions in LDL cholesterol and blood pressure through changes in diet and the early use of drugs were key preventive interventions. Reduced smoking, public availability of defibrillators, and an increased emphasis on exercise also contributed to the dramatic reduction in deaths from coronary artery disease.

These interventions were undertaken by individuals and organizations that shared the goal of reducing the devastating toll of coronary artery disease. The connections between these efforts, however, rarely went beyond shared goals.

Motor Vehicle Injuries

Deaths from motor vehicle injuries, especially automobiles, have also fallen dramatically in the last 75 years, especially when measured by deaths per mile driven. This impressive accomplishment required healthcare system, public health, and public policy interventions. These were each successful in their own right and reinforced the success in other components despite the fact that beyond shared goals, there were few connections between the components.

The healthcare system has contributed a well-functioning trauma system that has enabled many severely injured patients to walk out of the hospital. Public health interventions, from reducing the impact of alcohol to increasing the use of safety restraints, have played important roles in saving lives and reducing disability. Public policy interventions were required to set up and implement 911 and EMS systems and improve the safety of motor vehicles and roads.

Collaboration

In recent years, it has increasingly become evident that parallel play alone does not fully address our increasingly complex population health challenges. The movement toward more interprofessional education is an indicator of this need. The systems-doing strategy of collaboration is increasingly being used to address today's health challenges.

Active collaboration implies sharing more than goals. Collaboration implies that the components of the system share information, at least the essential information, and together develop a coherent set of plans to get the job done. The implementation of these plans may then be accomplished by each of the components of the system acting on its own.

Examples of successful collaboration include the following.

Spina Bifida and Other Neural Tube Defects

The number of children born with spina bifida and other neural tube defects has been reduced by approximately half in the last 25 years, and the impact on the affected children has been reduced. These efforts have included studies demonstrating that folic acid supplementation is very effective in preventing neural tube defects. Public health efforts to fortify the food supply have been particularly effective, though the quantity of fortification has been limited by the clinical concern that too much folic acid can mask the early signs of vitamin B-12 deficiency.

Screening for neuro-tube defects using sonography and maternal blood testing has provided early diagnosis. More recently, intrauterine surgery has shown signs of being an effective but costly intervention to reduce the consequences of neural tube defects.

All of these interventions connect as part of prenatal care. Collaboration now exists for prevention through folic acid supplementation, screening for early identification of neural tube defects, and immediate interventions after birth or intrauterine efforts to repair the defect.

Neurological Damage from Lead

Human exposure to lead goes back to ancient civilizations, yet in the 20th century, lead exposure dramatically increased with the use of lead to improve automobile performance and make paint apply better. By the 1970s, it was found that a large number of children in the United States had serum lead levels high enough to reduce intellectual ability.

Efforts to reduce lead levels in children required a collaborative effort between the healthcare system, public health, and public policy efforts. By the mid-1970s, there was a consensus that action needed to be taken. A key step was to phase out the use of lead in gasoline. This phaseout, however, was not completed until the mid-1990s. Thus, additional collaborative efforts were needed. Screening programs for serum lead were conducted as part of public health. Urban lands with high levels of lead were cleaned up before becoming children's playgrounds. Older homes were inspected for lead paint, and remedial efforts were supported by tax dollars.

The role of the healthcare system was primarily to educate and treat the most severely affected. Collaboration between the healthcare, public health, and social systems, while not perfect, has been key to reducing the exposure of children and improving the population's health.

These examples of collaboration remain the exception rather than the rule. Nonetheless, they are becoming more frequent with the increase in inter-professional education, digital technology for collaboration, and the increasing recognition of the importance of collaboration. The antibiotic resistance case study and the HIV case study at the end of this unit illustrate the ongoing challenges and importance of collaboration.

Integration of Efforts

At times, more than collaboration is needed to address complex problems; it requires integration of efforts. Integration of efforts implies more than planning together and selectively sharing information. It implies a joint implementation, often with a single organization or agency taking a lead role in implementation.

The types of challenges we face today include the potential for **pandemic** disease, such as influenza, and the ongoing need for disaster preparation and response. In both of these areas, it has been important to designate a lead agency and participating partners and create a flexible response system. We will call an approach to coordination that has all of these features the integration of efforts.

Examples of the developing utilization of integration of efforts include the following.

Disaster Prevention and Response

Disaster prevention and response have become important population health issues requiring an integrated approach. The lead integrative role increasingly being played by the Federal Emergency Management Administration (FEMA) has the potential to develop into an integrative model. The Hurricane Karl case study at the end of this unit illustrates the roles that the public health system and the healthcare system need to play in disaster prevention and response and the need for an integrative effort.

Influenza Pandemic

We have repeatedly faced the potential reality of new Influenza A strains and the potential for a worldwide epidemic or pandemic. No one agency or organization can address all the issues of coordination that are required to prevent and respond to the potential for another influenza pandemic, let alone the ongoing challenge of seasonal influenza that has killed 25,000 or more Americans in recent years.

TABLE 2-2 Models for Connecting the Components of the Health System

Approach to connecting	Meaning	Examples
Parallel play	▪ May share common goals, but work separately	Coronary artery disease, motor vehicle injuries, HIV, lung cancer
Collaboration	▪ Share common goals ▪ Coordinate planning and selective information sharing ▪ Separate implementation	Spina bifida, lead exposure, antibiotic resistance
Integration of efforts	▪ Share common goals ▪ Coordinated planning and full information sharing ▪ Joint implementation and evaluation	Disaster preparation and response, influenza

CDC in the United States and the World Health Organization (WHO) internationally play lead roles in the development of an integrated system of prevention and response. These efforts include the annual selection of influenza strains for inclusion in vaccines, the worldwide monitoring for new strains with potential for human-to-human spread, and the increasingly successful efforts to make vaccines accessible to everyone. These efforts require support and engagement from the healthcare system as well as the population at large. The influenza case study illustrates many of the challenges we face from the ongoing threat of pandemic influenza and new opportunities to improve vaccines.

TABLE 2-2 summarizes the three models for connecting the components of the health system that we have discussed.

Systems-doing, especially collaboration and integration of efforts, rarely occurs spontaneously. Experts are increasingly recognizing that institutional structures are needed to encourage systems-doing.

▶ What Institutional Structures Are Being Put in Place to Encourage Systems-Doing?

Efforts to implement a systems approach to population health are still in its early stages. **Community Health Needs Assessments** are being expanded as systems-thinking tools to improve population health.**

** The **Community-Oriented Primary Care (COPC)** movement represents an important precursor to the current approaches to community needs assessment and health impact assessment. COPC is focused on how community health organizations can address the needs of the community as well as the needs of individuals. COPC uses a structured process to define and characterize a community and prioritize its health needs.

Community Health Needs Assessment is a systematic examination of the health status indicators for a given population used to identify key problems and assets in a community. The ultimate goal of a community health assessment is to develop strategies to address the community's health needs and identified issues.[20]

Community Health Needs Assessments are increasingly becoming a mechanism for encouraging coordination between the public health and healthcare systems. The Patient Protection and Affordable Care Act (ACA) now requires hospitals to regularly conduct community health assessments. Public health agencies are also required to conduct a form of a Community Health Needs Assessment as part of a new voluntary accreditation process by the Public Health Accreditation Board.[21]

The results of a community health assessment might look something like this: a Community Health Assessment was conducted in a large Hispanic/Latino community defined by census tracks. The vast majority of the community is employed, and over half of the working population receive minimum wage and have no health insurance. There are a large number of immigrants from Central America. Over 25% of the community is estimated to be undocumented aliens, most of whom live in crowded conditions. A high percentage of those over 18 are married with an average family size of 5—considerably larger than other communities in the same city. The population of the community is generally younger than the surrounding, more affluent communities. The vast majority of the community receives its health care at one community clinic.

In addition to collecting data on the availability of health services and the causes of death and disability, a sample of community residents were asked about what they saw as their most important health priorities. The community's priority issues included TB, HIV/AIDS, a lack of recreational facilities for children, a lack of dental services, and a lack of Spanish-speaking healthcare professionals. Health care and public health professionals saw TB, HIV/AIDS as their top priority, while the community considered lack of dental care their #1 priority.

Community Health Needs Assessments have the potential to increase collaboration between hospitals and health systems with local health departments to accomplish the expectations of Community Health Assessments.[††]

As we have seen, systems-thinking has become a foundational framework for population health, along with a population health perspective. Systems-thinking is a six-step process for analyzing problems leading to identification of bottlenecks and leverage points when interventions can be especially effective.

---

†† Community Health Assessments do not themselves guarantee collaborative interventions. A second, new initiative known as **Health Impact Assessment** is increasingly being used to bring together the health system with other systems that impact health, from housing to transportation to education. According to the CDC, a Health Impact Assessment (HIA) is a process that helps evaluate the potential health effects of a plan, project, or policy before it is built or implemented. HIA brings potential positive and negative public health impacts and considerations to the decision-making process for plans, projects, and policies that fall outside traditional public health arenas, such as transportation and land use. An HIA provides practical recommendations to increase positive health effects and minimize negative health effects.[22]

Successful efforts to meet the complicated challenges we face require us to do more than systems-thinking; we need systems-doing. Systems-doing is built on mutual knowledge of the roles played by each component of the system and coordination of components of the larger health system to be sure that they function effectively together. We have looked at three types of coordination: parallel play, collaboration, and integration of efforts.

Population health requires us to utilize both systems-thinking and systems-doing. Together, these approaches hold great promise for bringing together health care, public health, as well as public policy interventions to improve the population's health.

🔍 CASE STUDIES AND DISCUSSION QUESTIONS

HIV/AIDS: A Population Health History

Discussion Questions
Return to the HIV/AIDS case study in the introduction and discuss the following:

1. How are the following features of systems-thinking illustrated in the case of HIV/AIDS?
   - Connections between components, i.e., health care, public health, public policy intervention
   - Interactions between diseases
   - Bottlenecks and leverage points
2. What type(s) of systems-doing is/are illustrated in the case of HIV/AIDS?

Lung Cancer: Old Disease, New Approaches
Lung cancer in the United States today is the most commonly diagnosed life-threatening cancer among both men and women, with over 150,000 deaths per year. Cases of lung cancer increase with advancing age, with the disease rarely occurring before age 50. Lung cancer is usually diagnosed at a late stage. The duration of the disease after diagnosis is often measured in months, and the chance of death within a year or two after the diagnosis is made is well above 90%.

Cigarette smoking has been recognized as the most important contributory cause of lung cancer since 1964, when the data were sufficient for the U.S. surgeon general to publish the first of a series of reports on smoking and health, concluding that cigarette smoking is a cause of lung cancer and that interventions are needed to reduce the rate of cigarette smoking.

A large number of specific interventions have been studied and implemented, many with some success. Nearly 50% of men and 25% of women smoked cigarettes in the United States in the early 1960s. Initial efforts to reduce smoking included public service announcements and warning labels on cigarettes. The rate of smoking in the 1960s modestly reduced among men, but little or no change occurred among women. In fact, over the subsequent decades, the rates of cigarette smoking increased among young women. During these years, tobacco

(continues)

🔎 CASE STUDIES AND DISCUSSION QUESTIONS *(continued)*

companies advertised Virginia Slims and other products, which associated smoking with weight loss and may have led to increased smoking among young women.

During the 1980s and early 1990s, efforts included increased taxes on cigarettes and restrictions of cigarette smoking in public places, including airplanes and increasingly in the workplace justified by evidence of the hazards of second-hand smoking. Evaluation efforts indicated a gradual reduction in smoking, with rates falling to less than 25% among both adult men and women.

However, the evaluation data indicated that the rates among adolescents were increasing to above 35% by the mid-1990s. In addition, it was recognized that nearly 90% of adult smokers began smoking before age 18 and most at a much earlier age. This led to a better understanding of the addictive nature of smoking and the need for interventions aimed at preventing addiction and addressing it through behavioral modification and drug treatments.

By the late 1990s, efforts were directed at reducing the rate of smoking among adolescents. A range of interventions were introduced. Peer education, even higher taxes on cigarettes, and laws preventing advertising of cigarettes and selling cigarettes to minors, such as the Joe Camel campaign, were among the interventions used. The subsequent rates of cigarette smoking among adolescents gradually fell to approximately the same rates as those of adults.

Data suggest that most of the 15%–20% of the population who continue to smoke are strongly addicted to nicotine and that education and even motivation are not likely to be effective. Recent efforts have turned to the regulation of nicotine in cigarettes, and the FDA now has the authority to regulate but not eliminate nicotine in cigarettes.

Pregnant women have been recognized as a group who are highly motivated to stop smoking to prevent the adverse effects on their offspring. Efforts to stop smoking during pregnancy have the potential to carry over beyond delivery. Early detection, extra attention, and insurance coverage for cessation efforts have become widespread strategies for addressing smoking during pregnancy.

The declining rate of cigarette smoking in the United States has been coupled with a better recognition of other factors that play roles in the development of lung cancer today. A large number of Americans have been exposed to asbestos, a substance used as insulation in building, in brake linings, and in many other applications. It was widely used in the shipbuilding industry during World War II, where several million workers were heavily exposed. Restrictions on the use of asbestos and regulations of renovation and demolition of asbestos-containing buildings have greatly reduced exposures to asbestos.

Uranium miners in several countries have been found to have an increased risk of developing lung cancer even in the absence of cigarette smoking. Radon, a naturally occurring invisible, odorless gas that is produced by the breakdown of uranium, was found to be widely present in homes in many geographic areas not just those with uranium mines. Investigators began to examine whether there was a connection between radon gas exposure and lung cancer.

Approximately 20,000 cases of lung cancer per year are now attributed to radon exposure by the Environmental Protection Agency. About 1 in 15 homes currently have radon exposures above the levels at which the Environmental Protection Agency recommends action. The EPA recommends voluntary routine home testing. However, the major effort to successfully control radon exposure has been introducing laws requiring testing prior to sale of a property and compulsory reductions in levels when high levels are detected.

The importance of asbestos and radon exposures has been apparent based on data indicating that these risk factors for lung cancer have multiplicative effects on the risk when combined with cigarette smoking. For instance, when the relative risk of asbestos is 5 and the relative risk of cigarette smoking is 10, the risk when there is exposure to both is nearly 50. Thus, reductions in either of these risk factors can have dramatic impacts on the overall risk of lung cancer among those who also smoke cigarettes.

Early detection and treatment of lung cancer by chest X-rays have been shown to have little, if any, impact. Studies of routine chest X-rays for long-term smokers have been shown to produce a slightly earlier diagnosis, but to merely extend the time between diagnosis and death. Once evident on chest X-ray, the lung cancer is nearly always beyond the point of cure.

Recent studies have confirmed that a newer type of X-ray test, called a spiral computerized tomogram, or spiral CT, is capable of diagnosing lung cancer at an earlier stage. The test is expensive and has **false positives** as well as **false negatives**. However, it has been shown to modestly reduce the deaths due to lung cancer. Controversy continues over when to use spiral CT for screening for lung cancer.

An appreciation of the causes of lung cancer has led to multiple efforts to reduce exposure and detect and treat it early. The incidence rates of lung cancer in recent years have begun to fall, but the disease remains the most common cause of cancer deaths in both men and women. Increasingly, a systems-thinking approach is being used to develop a coherent approach to reducing the incidence rate and the mortality rate due to lung cancer.

Discussion Questions
1. How was systems-thinking used to identify multiple factors and investigate their interactions, as illustrated in this case? Explain.
2. How was systems-thinking used to identify bottlenecks and leverage points, as illustrated in this case? Explain.
3. How would you combine the strategies discussed in this case to address the issue of lung cancer? Explain.
4. What systems-doing approach(es) would you use to implement the strategies you have identified for addressing the issue of lung cancer? Explain.

Antibiotic Resistance: It's with Us for the Long Run
It was too good to be true: when penicillin was first introduced in clinical practice during World War II, it had dramatic impacts on a range of infectious diseases, from pneumococcal pneumonia, to gonorrhea, to staphylococcal wound infections.

(continues)

🔍 *CASE STUDIES AND DISCUSSION QUESTIONS* *(continued)*

No randomized controlled trials were needed to demonstrate its efficacy or effectiveness compared with previous treatments. In short order, however, higher dosages of penicillin were required, and by the early 1950s, penicillin stopped working altogether for many infections.

In the 1950s, new classes of antibiotics were developed, which headed off a crisis. However, it was already apparent that bacteria had the ability to develop resistance to antibiotics using a range of mechanisms. The more aggressively antibiotics were used, the more common resistance became, especially in hospitals where antibiotics had literally become standard operating procedure.

In addition to the use of antibiotics to treat bacterial infections, it became common clinical practice to try antibiotics as a first-line approach when the cause of the problem was not clear or was most likely due to a virus. In addition, it was found that antibiotics could modestly increase the growth rate of many animals raised for food. Widespread use of antibiotics in farm animals allowed the development of feedlots and whole industries devoted to raising animals together in close quarters.

By the late 20th century, animal use of antibiotics exceeded human use. These antibiotics often ended up in public water systems, where the runoff from feedlots contaminates streams and groundwater. It has been called a "double hit." We got antibiotics in our food and in our drinking water, both of which promote bacterial resistance.

By the early years of this century, the problem of antibiotic resistance returned with a vengeance. Methicillin-resistant *Staphylococcus aureus* infections, or MRSA, became widespread not only in hospitals, but in the community as well. Healthy athletes as well as those undergoing outpatient surgeries were now at risk of life-threatening diseases. Community-acquired MRSA skin infections are increasingly common in groups that share close quarters or experience more skin-to-skin contact, such as team athletes, military recruits, and prisoners. However, MRSA infections are being seen in the general community as well, including in individuals without known risk factors.

The problem is broader than staphylococcal infection; in fact, the vast majority of bacteria that causes infections in hospitals are resistant to at least one of the antibiotics previously used for their treatment. Recently, gram-negative infections, which are the most common causes of urinary tract infections and an increasingly frequent cause of pneumonia and postsurgical infections, have often become resistant to multiple antibiotics. The CDC estimates that over 20,000 people per year die in the United States alone from antibiotic-resistant bacterial infections.

Reducing the consequences of the existing antibiotic resistance is critical. Increased hand-washing and use of other sterilizing procedures is underway in healthcare institutions. Parallel precautions might be needed in athletic and fitness facilities. Early nonantibiotic treatments of wounds and other acute conditions is becoming an important intervention.

Previously unrecognized impacts of overuse of antibiotics are increasingly being recognized. These are likely to include increases in childhood asthma and juvenile idiopathic arthritis. There is even suggestive evidence of an increase in childhood obesity associated with early use of antibiotics. These previously unexpected impacts are all being linked to changes in the human microbiome that are due to overuse of antibiotics. The human microbiome consists of billions of bacteria and other microbes that live outside and inside all human beings, most commonly in the gastrointestinal tract.

In recent years, routine feeding of antibiotics to animals has been banned in much of the developed world and is now being curtailed in the United States. New approaches to reducing the development and spread of antibiotic-resistant bacteria are underway, and new classes of antibiotics are under investigation. Before clinical use, they will need FDA approval. Once approved, the FDA will need to decide whether they should be available for all licensed prescribers or restricted to specifically qualified prescribers and/or specific conditions/diseases.

Alternative or complementary approaches, such as greater reliance on vaccinations, may reduce the need for antibiotics. For instance, vaccines to prevent pneumococcal and meningococcal bacterial disease have been highly successful. Use of nonprescription probiotics, or "good bacteria," has been shown to improve the tolerance for, and at times the effectiveness of, existing antibiotics. They are increasingly being used as a routine adjunct to treatment and possibly for prevention.

New approaches to antibiotic resistance may come from the rapidly expanding understanding of the relationship between human health, animal health, and ecosystem health. The issue of antibiotic resistance to treatment is not new, and it is not going away.

Discussion Questions

1. What aspects of One Health and systems-thinking are illustrated in this case study?
2. If a new class of antibiotics is developed and approved by the FDA, what type of restrictions should be placed on its use, if any? Explain.
3. What interventions do you recommend for reducing the impact of bacteria that are already resistant to multiple antibiotics? Explain.
4. How should the recently recognized impacts of antibiotic overuse affect recommendations for use of antibiotics in primary care practice? Explain.

Hurricane Karl and the Public Health Success in Old Orleans

Hurricane Karl, a category four hurricane, made landfall last August 29 on the gold coast of the state of Good Fortune. The state is home to the town of Old Orleans, a historical community built below sea level and home to a large community from a range of socioeconomic backgrounds. Old Orleans has a model health department that seeks to provide the 10 essential public health services.

Before Hurricane Karl made its impact on the community, preparation for hurricanes had been an ongoing activity of the health department. The health department took the lead as part of a Disaster Preparation Task Force, which worked closely with first responders to ensure safe evacuation and protection from fire and looting. In its role leading the Task Force, The Health Department also worked with local TV and radio stations to advise citizens on the purchasing and storing of essential food, water, and first aid supplies. It

(continues)

organized a community-wide emergency care network to ensure that 911 calls were responded to as quickly as possible in the event of a hurricane and worked with local hospitals to ensure that a triage system was in place to allocate patients to available emergency facilities, while not overwhelming any one healthcare institution.

When Hurricane Karl did strike, the damage was more extensive than expected. Leaks in the public sewer system led to water contamination. A local chemical plant experienced a major chemical discharge. Almost 200 residents were stranded in their homes without adequate food. Nearly half of the homes experienced water damage and rapid growth of mold. Many older residents did not have access to their daily medications.

The local health department had prepared for disasters like Hurricane Karl. After testing the water for contamination, supplies of stockpiled bottled water were distributed to homes in the contaminated areas by the National Guard. The police department had purchased specially equipped vehicles on the recommendation of the health department and was able, with the help of community organizations, to evacuate the stranded residents.

The health department also sent out trained teams to diagnose the type and extent of hazards related to chemical contamination. With the help of the emergency radio system and cell phones, all individuals in the contaminated areas were notified and educated about methods for protecting themselves and their children.

Based on the emergency plan, the health department set up temporary healthcare sites and pharmacies staffed by nurses, physicians, and pharmacists who had been certified as emergency responders. The department also worked with representatives of the building industry to test water-exposed homes for mold and provided assistance to minimize the damage.

After the emergency, the health department joined with the local schools of public health and medicine to evaluate the response to Hurricane Karl and make recommendations for future emergencies. The data on infections, injuries, and deaths, as well as the use of services during the emergency, were collected and published. A national network was set up as a result to coordinate efforts for future disasters and learn from the experience in dealing with Hurricane Karl.

Discussion Questions

1. Which of the 10 essential services did the health department of Old Orleans fulfill? Explain.
2. What efforts beyond those of the health department were needed to accomplish the 10 essential public health services? Explain.
3. In addition to providing the 10 essential public health services, what efforts are required to deal with a disaster such as Hurricane Karl? Explain.
4. What type of systems-doing is illustrated in this case, i.e., parallel play, collaboration, integration? Explain.

References

1. Merriam-Webster. System. http://www.merriam-webster.com/dictionary/system. Accessed June 15, 2018.
2. O'Connor J, McDermott I. *The Art of Systems Thinking: Essential Skills for Creativity and Problem Solving.* Phoenix, AZ: Premium Source Publishing; 2006.
3. The Open University. Systems thinking and practice: Diagramming. http://systems.open .ac.uk/materials/T552. Accessed June 15, 2018.
4. Institute of Medicine. The healthcare imperative: lowering costs and improving outcomes-workshop series summary. https://www.nap.edu/catalog/12750/the-healthcare-imperative -lowering-costs-and-improving-outcomes-workshop-series. Accessed July 16, 2018.
5. U.S. Food and Drug Administration. Hazard analysis & critical control points (HACCP). http://www.fda.gov/Food/Guidanceregulation/HACCP. Accessed June 15, 2018.
6. Kohn LT, Corrigan JM, Donaldson MS, eds. *To Err Is Human: Building a Safer Health System.* Vol. 6. Washington, DC: National Academies Press; 2000.
7. Institute of Medicine Committee on Quality of Care in America. *Crossing the Quality Chasm: A New Health System for the 21st Century.* Washington, DC: National Academy Press; 2001.
8. Patient Safety Movement. Actionable patient safety solutions. Creating a culture of safety. http://patientsafetymovement.org/challenge/creating-a-culture-of-safety/. Accessed June 15, 2018.
9. Barach P, Small SD. Reporting and preventing medical mishaps: lessons from non-medical near miss reporting systems. *Br Med J.* 2000;320(7237):759–763.
10. One Health Initiative. About the One Health Initiative. http://www.onehealthinitiative.com /about.php. Accessed June 15, 2018.
11. Woolhouse MEJ, Adair K, Brierley L. RNA viruses: a case study of the biology of emerging infectious diseases. *Microbiol Spectr.* 2013;1(1). doi:10.1128/microbiolspec.OH-0001-2012.
12. Morse SS. Factors in the emergence of infectious diseases. *Emerging Infectious Diseases.* January 1995. http://wwwnc.cdc.gov/eid/article/1/1/95-0102. Accessed June 15, 2018.
13. Crimmins A, Balbus JL, Gamble CB, et al. Executive summary. In: *The Impacts of Climate Change on Human Health in the United States: A Scientific Assessment.* Washington, DC: U.S. Global Change Research Program; 2016: 1–24. http://dx.doi.org/10.7930/J0OP0WXS.
14. National Institutes of Health. Can pets help keep you healthy? NIH News in Health. February 2009:1–2. https://newsinhealth.nih.gov/2009/February/feature1.htm. Accessed July 26, 2017.
15. Centers for Disease Control and Prevention. Parasites-toxoplasmosis. http://www.cdc.gov /parasites/toxoplasmosis. Accessed June 15, 2018.
16. Centers for Disease Control and Prevention. Cat-scratch disease. http://www.cdc.gov /healthypets/diseases/cat-scratch.html. Accessed June 15, 2018.
17. Centers for Disease Control and Prevention. Parasites-toxocariasis (also known as Roundworm Infection). http://www.cdc.gov/parasites/toxocariasis/. Accessed June 15, 2018.
18. Families USA. 10 Essential health benefits insurance plans must cover under the affordable care act. https://familiesusa.org/blog/10-essential-health-benefits-insurance-plans-must-cover Accessed July 2, 2018.
19. The Public Health System and the 10 Essential Public Health Services. https://www.cdc.gov /stltpublichealth/publichealthservices/essentialhealthservices.html. Accessed June 15, 2018.
20. Turnock B. *Public Health: What It Is and How It Works.* Sudbury, MA: Jones & Bartlett Publishers 2009.
21. Public Health Accreditation Board. Getting started. http://www.phaboard.org/accreditation -overview/getting-started/. Accessed June 15, 2018.
22. Centers for Disease Control and Prevention. Health impact assessment. https://www.cdc.gov /healthyplaces/hia.htm. Accessed June 15, 2018.

UNIT 3

Tools of Population Health

LEARNING OBJECTIVES

By the end of this unit, students will be able to:

- Identify the types of data used in population health
- Describe implementation strategies used in population health
- Describe the uses of health communications in population health
- Describe the role of population health in producing behavioral change
- Describe the role of health policy interventions in population health
- Describe the role of screening for disease and risk factors in population health
- Describe the role of population-based vaccination in disease eradication and control

The tools of population health represent the third foundational framework of population health. They build upon and grow out of the population health framework and the systems-thinking/systems-doing framework. Underpinning the tools of population health is the data that provide evidence for the selection of interventions to address population health problems.

Evidence in population health comes from a range of sources, both qualitative and quantitative, including the following:

- Surveillance: Continuous collection of data, including births and deaths, reportable diseases, as well as adverse effects of drugs and vaccines. Surveillance also includes active data collection for special purposes, ranging from antibiotic resistance to birth defects, to early detection of influenza A.
- Surveys: Health care, public health, and public policy surveys range from hospital discharge data to regularly conducted population surveys for health and nutrition, to census data.
- Studies: Investigations designed to establish causation and the efficacy of interventions, including **case–control studies**, **cohort studies**, and **randomized**

controlled trials, as well as investigations that evaluate the effectiveness and safety of interventions in practice.

■ Synthesis: Evidence synthesis includes systematic reviews, which comprehensively collect and synthesize all available quantitative and qualitative data on a topic and meta-analysis that aims to quantitatively combine and analyze peer-reviewed literature on a specific issue.

Evidence forms the basis for explanation leading to evidence-based problem solving and prediction leading to evidence-based decision-making. Together, these types of evidence form the basis for selection of the tools to be used to improve population health. To better understand this process, let's look at the basic strategies used in population health, followed by a look at key tools for implementation in population health.

▶ What Are the Basic Strategies for Improving Population Health?

There are three basic strategies used to improve population health. We will categorize them as follows:

■ **Reducing high risk**
■ **Improving the average risk**
■ **Narrowing the spread of the risk curve**

The "reducing high risk" strategy focuses on those with the highest probability of developing disease and aims to bring their risk closer to the levels experienced by the rest of the population. **FIGURE 3-1** demonstrates the "reducing high risk" strategy.

The success of the "reducing high risk" strategy assumes that those with a high probability of developing disease are heavily concentrated among those with exposure to known risk factors. Risk factors include a wide range of exposures, from cigarette smoke and other toxic substances to high-risk sexual behaviors. Strategies aimed at high-risk individuals often utilize the healthcare system to identify and attempt to reduce the risk. Traditional public health and public policy interventions may be useful to support or complement these efforts.

The "improving the average risk" strategy focuses on the entire population and aims to reduce the risk for everyone. **FIGURE 3-2** illustrates this strategy.

The "improving the average risk" strategy assumes that a large proportion of a population is at some degree of risk, and the risk increases with the extent of exposure.* In this situation, most of the disease occurs among the large number of people who have only modestly increased exposure. The successful reduction in average cholesterol levels through changes in the U.S. diet and the anticipated reduction in diabetes via a focus on weight reduction among children illustrate

---

* This assumes, as is often the situation, that the distribution of a risk factor is bell shaped or normally distributed. In this situation, there is a large number of individuals with only modestly elevated risk who are often the ones who experience a large proportion of the adverse outcomes.

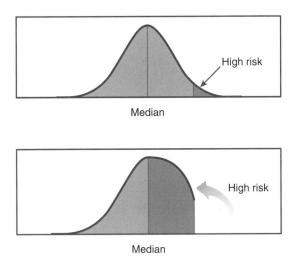

FIGURE 3-1 (A) High Risk and (B) Reducing High Risk

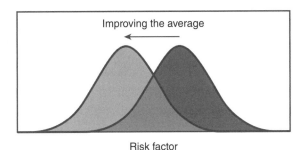

FIGURE 3-2 Improving the Average

this strategy. Strategies aimed at improving the average often rely on traditional public health and public policy interventions, with health care helping to reinforce their efforts.

A final strategy that may be used occasionally is narrowing the spread of the risk curve, as illustrated in **FIGURE 3-3**. This strategy may require an increase in the risk for low-risk groups while reducing the risk for high-risk groups. This strategy relies primarily on public policy interventions. Efforts to reduce air pollution in high-risk urban neighborhoods by building higher industrial smoke stacks was an unsuccessful way to reduce exposure in high-risk neighborhoods by increasing exposure downwind in low-risk exposure communities. Efforts to increase taxes on the wealthy to pay for increased health services for those who cannot afford health insurance may also be seen as utilizing the "narrowing the spread of the risk curve" strategy. It is built on the assumption that a large gain for the currently uninsured will have only modest impacts on the currently insured.

Therefore, population health has at its disposal a range of strategies that can be used alone or in combination to improve the health of the public. There are some key tools

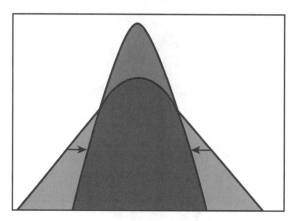

FIGURE 3-3 Narrowing the Spread of the Risk Curve

that are unique to population health. We will examine five tools of population health, which together we will call the third foundational framework of population health.

This third foundational framework of population health includes the following tools of the trade:

- Population health communications
- Population-based behavioral change
- Health policy interventions
- Screening for disease and risk factors for disease
- Population-based vaccination for disease eradication and control

Let's look at each of these tools of population health.

▶ **What Is Population Health Communications?**

Health communications is an exploding field that is developing faster than the speed of the Internet. All components of the health system increasingly rely on electronic communications, including the Internet and its nearly unlimited capacity.

Population health increasingly relies on health communications through mass media, especially the Internet, including social media. Population health has begun to apply marketing approaches to health education as well as to understanding and changing health behavior. **Social marketing**, a use and extension of traditional product marketing, has become a key tool of population health.[1]

Social marketing campaigns were first successfully used in the developing world to promote a range of products and behaviors, including family planning and pediatric rehydration therapy. In recent years, social marketing efforts have been widely and successfully used in developed countries, including efforts such as the following:

- The truth® campaign: Developed by the American Legacy Foundation, it aims to redirect the perception of smoking from being seen as a teenage rebellion to the decision to not smoke being a rebellion against the alleged behavior-controlling tobacco industry.

- The National Youth Anti-Drug campaign: It uses social marketing efforts directed at young people, including the "Parents. The Anti-Drug." campaign.
- The VERB™ campaign: It focuses on 9- to 13-year-olds, or "tweens," with a goal of making exercise fun and "cool" for everyone, not just competitive athletes.

Social marketing efforts in developing and developed countries have demonstrated that it is possible to change key health behaviors of well-defined groups of people, including adolescents, who are often regarded as the hardest to reach. An example of the use of social marketing to reach young people, the VERB™ campaign, is examined in **BOX 3-1**.[2]

To be successful, social marketing needs to address a series of questions[3]:

1. What is the goal?
2. Who has power over the goal?
3. To whom do individuals listen?
4. How can you get the message across to them?
5. How can you effectively put forward the message?

It is important to see the development of messages as only one part of effective communication. The development of a consistent and engaging message is a key component of all population health communications. A useful framework for

BOX 3-1 VERB™ Campaign

The VERB™ social marketing campaign was funded through the Centers for Disease Control and Prevention (CDC), which worked with advertising agencies to reach tweens and make exercise "cool." After a series of focus groups and other efforts to define and understand the market, it was concluded that the message should not be one of improving health, but rather of having fun with friends, exploring new activities with a sense of adventure, and being free to experiment without being judged on performance.

Marketing efforts also identified barriers, including time constraints and the attraction of other activities, from social occasions to television to computers. In addition, barriers included lack of access to facilities as well as negative images of competition, embarrassment, and the inability to become an elite athlete.

The VERB™ campaign implied action and used the tagline "It's what you do." Initial messages used animated figures of children covered with verbs being physically active. Later, messages turned these animated verb-covered kids into real kids playing actively. Widely used logos were developed and promoted as part of the branding effort. The VERB™ campaign partnered with television channels that successfully reach tweens, sponsored outreach events, and distributed promotional materials.

During the 4 years of the VERB™ campaign, tweens developed widespread recognition of the program and rated it highly in terms of "saying something important to me" (64%) and "makes me want to get more active" (68%).

Data from Wong F, Huhman M, Asbury L, Mueller RB, McCarthy S, Londe P, et al. VERB™—A social marketing campaign to increase physical activity among youth. *Prev Chronic Disease*. 2004;3(1):1–7.

messaging has been called the SUCCESs framework.[4] The components of the SUC-CESs framework are:

- Simplicity
- Unexpectedness
- Concreteness
- Credibility
- Emotions
- Stories

Few efforts at population health communications satisfy all of these criteria for success. However, having set criteria lets us judge how much we fall short. Let's take a look at an example of a highly successful population health intervention that relies heavily on population health communications, i.e., the Back-to-Sleep campaign to reduce SIDS.

TABLE 3-1 outlines the use of the SUCCESs framework as applied to the Back-to-Sleep campaign, which has greatly contributed to reducing SIDS deaths in the United States by approximately 50%.

Health communications underpin the effectiveness of the other tools of population health that we will address. It overlaps and is an essential component of the next tool we will explore, which is population-based behavioral change.

TABLE 3-1 SUCCESs in Public Health Communication: The Back-To-Sleep Campaign

Element	Meaning	SIDS Back-to-Sleep campaign
Simplicity	Being able to capture meaning in a few words	Three words, Back-to-Sleep, capture the meaning
Unexpectedness	Getting and holding people's attention	Catchy and easy to remember
Concreteness	Easily visualizable	Says what should be done
Credibility	Can be reinforced by trustworthy sources of information	Clinicians, caregivers, and even crib retailers can reinforce
Emotions	Connect to emotions; assists in gaining attention and remembering	Alludes to the ability to prevent infant deaths
Stories	Short personalized stories are easily recalled	Suffocation for infants who can't roll over is an easy-to-imagine story

Data from Heath C, Heath D. *Made to Stick: Why Some Ideas Survive and Others Die.* New York: Random House; 2007.

▶ What Do We Mean by Population-Based Behavioral Change?

A great deal of the success of population health depends on successful efforts to change individual behavior. Whether we are talking about obesity, opioid use, cigarette smoking, seat belt use, safer sex, vaccination, obtaining a mammogram, improving nutrition, or increasing exercise, etc., human behavior is at the center of population health.

Human behavior is often considered an inherently individual action. Nonetheless, population-based influences have strong impacts on how individuals behave. We often use the term "**culture**" to describe the multiple economic, religious, and habitual influences on the actions of large numbers of people.

Culture, in a broad sense, helps people make judgments about the world and decisions about behavior. Culture defines what is good or bad and what is healthy or unhealthy. This may relate to lifestyle patterns, beliefs about risk, and beliefs about body type; for example, a large body type in some cultures symbolizes health, prosperity, and well-being, not obesity, high risk, or other negative implications.

Culture directly affects the daily habits of life. Food choice and methods of food preparation and preservation are all affected by culture as well as socioeconomic status. For instance, the Mediterranean diet, which includes olive oil, seafood, vegetables, nuts, and fruits, has been shown to have benefits for the heart even when used in countries far removed from the Mediterranean.

There are often clear-cut negative and/or positive impacts on disability related to cultural traditions as diverse as feet binding in China and female genital mutilation in some parts of Africa. Some societies reject strenuous physical activity for those who have the status and wealth to be served by others.

Culture is also related to an individual's response to symptoms and acceptance of interventions. In many cultures, medical care is exclusively for those with symptoms and is not part of prevention. Many traditional cultures have developed sophisticated systems of self-care and self-medication supported by family and traditional healers. These traditions greatly affect how individuals respond to symptoms, how they communicate the symptoms, and the types of medical and public health interventions that they will accept. Thus, culture, a population concept, is closely tied to the behavior of individuals and needs to be understood in order to change behavior as part of improving population health. **TABLE 3-2** outlines a range of ways in which culture can affect health.

A widely used theory of behavioral change is known as the **Stages of Change model**. The Stages of Change model states that individuals go through a series of changes when making and maintaining behavioral change. Let's examine these phases and then see how individual- and population-based behavioral changes are needed using the example of cigarette cessation.

The stages of change are as follows:

Precontemplation: The first stage, called precontemplation, implies that an individual has not yet considered changing his or her behavior. At this stage, efforts to encourage change are not likely to be successful. However, efforts to educate and offer help in the future may lay the groundwork for later success.

TABLE 3-2 Examples of Ways That Culture Can Affect Health	
Ways that culture may affect health	**Examples**
Culture is related to behavior—social practices may put individuals and groups at increased or reduced risk	Food preferences—vegetarian Mediterranean diet Cooking methods History of binding of feet in China Female genital mutilation Role of exercise
Culture is related to response to symptoms, such as the level of urgency to recognize symptoms, seek care, and communicate symptoms	Cultural differences in seeking care and self-medication Social, family, and work structures provide varying degrees of social support—low degree of social support may be associated with reduced health-related quality of life
Culture is related to the types of interventions that are acceptable	Variations in degree of acceptance of traditional Western medicine, including reliance on self-help and traditional healers
Culture is related to the response to disease and interventions	Cultural differences in follow-up, adherence to treatment, and acceptance of adverse outcome

Contemplation: The second phase, known as contemplation, implies that an individual is actively thinking about the benefits and barriers to change. At this stage, information focused on short- and immediate-term gains, as well as long-term benefits, can be especially useful. In addition, the contemplation stage lends itself to developing a baseline—that is, establishing the current severity or extent of the problem in order to measure future progress.

Preparation: The third phase is called preparation. During this phase, the individual is developing a plan of action. At this point, the individual may be especially receptive to setting goals, considering a range of strategies, and developing a timetable. Help in recognizing and preparing for unanticipated barriers can be especially useful to the individual during this phase.

Action: The fourth phase is the action phase, when the change in behavior takes place. This is the time to bring together all possible outside support to reinforce and reward the new behavior and help with problems or setbacks that occur.

Maintenance: The fifth—and hopefully final—phase is the maintenance phase, in which the new behavior becomes a permanent part of an individual's lifestyle. The maintenance phase requires education on how to anticipate the long-term nature of

TABLE 3-3 Stages of Change: Individual, Group, and Population/Social Interventions to Change Cigarette Smoking Behavior

Stage of change	Individual interventions	Population health interventions
Precontemplation	Assess readiness for change and offer future help	Social marketing aimed at specific groups; restriction on smoking at work and public places; vivid and changing label on cigarette packages
Contemplation	Information on hazards of smoking and gains from quitting	Focus on taxation and the cost of cigarettes as incentive to quit.
Preparation	Set individual goals, and develop strategy Medication may be helpful	Telephone "quit hotline" for information and encouragement Population health process of approving drugs and monitoring drug safety
Action	Remove connections between cigarettes and pleasurable activities, use of medications if needed	National efforts, e.g., American Cancer Society national quit day Insurance coverage for smoking cessation programs and medications
Maintenance	Education regarding long-term physical addiction and potential for relapse	Continued reinforcement by social marketing, taxes, and restriction on smoking

behavioral change, especially how to resist the inevitable temptations to resume the old behavior.

Population health interventions are key to each of these stages. To be successful, individual and population-based interventions need to reinforce each other. **TABLE 3-3** outlines ways in which population health can play a role in each of the stages of behavioral change for cigarette cessation efforts.

Population-based behavioral change and other population health interventions usually require supportive health policies to provide guiderails and incentives for behaviors, or "carrots and sticks." Health policies and laws that support tobacco reduction range from restriction on smoking to regulation of nicotine in cigarettes and from taxation of cigarettes to insurance coverage for smoking cessation efforts. Let's take a broader look at how health policies can be used to improve population health.

▶ How Can Health Policies Be Used to Improve Population Health?

Health policies result from federal, state, and local legislation as well as from executive branch action. They also include private actions by employers, health insurance corporations, and healthcare providers that influence what individuals can and cannot do. For instance, with cigarette cessation, important health policies include but are not limited to the following:

- FDA legislative authority to regulate nicotine in cigarettes
- FDA approval of drugs for smoking cessation and monitoring for safety
- Subsidies for tobacco farmers to encourage or discourage tobacco production
- Local and state bans on smoking in indoor public areas, including bars and restaurants
- Insurance coverage for smoking cessation programs and medications
- Employers' decision to prohibit cigarette smoking at work
- Healthcare organizations' no smoking policies.

In recent years, two important population health approaches to health policies have emerged that are likely to grow in importance in the coming years. These are as follows:

- Global action to address health conditions that cross national borders, such as pandemic disease
- Health-in-all-policies that view health as a single system.

Let's look at these two population health approaches to health policy.

Global Action to Address Health Conditions That Cross National Borders Such as Pandemic Disease

Pandemic disease requires more than a national response; it requires a global response. Epidemic and widespread pandemics have occurred since ancient times, yet until recently, there was little coordinated international response.

World Health Organization (WHO) was established as a United Nations organization in 1948. In 1951, WHO adopted the **International Health Regulations** (IHR), which became binding for all WHO members. These regulations were initially limited to cholera, plague, yellow fever, and smallpox, with smallpox being removed after its eradication in the late 1970s.

Severe threats to global health occurred before the international community succeeded in modernizing the IHR. In 2005, after the SARS epidemic, the IHR were modified in a number of important ways.[5,6]

The scope of the IHR (2005) was expanded with an aim to prevent, protect against, control, and provide a public health response to the international spread of disease.

- The IHR (2005) embraced an all-hazards strategy, covering health threats irrespective of their origin or source as opposed to the previous disease-specific coverage. The intention was to include biological, chemical, and nuclear events, etc.
- The IHR (2005) require nations to develop "core capacities" for rapid detection, assessment, reporting, and response to potential **public health emergencies**

of international concern, including for surveillance, laboratories, and risk communication. Core capacities were central to a population health strategy of strengthening local infrastructure and systems to detect and contain outbreaks at their source before they spread internationally.

- To be in compliance, member countries were required to promptly notify WHO of events that might constitute a public health emergency of international concern (PHEIC), with a continuing obligation to inform WHO of any updates.
- On the basis of information from nations (official sources) and/or from unofficial sources, WHO's Director General was authorized to declare what is called a "public health emergency of international concern." Declaration of a PHEIC allowed WHO to make unbinding disease control recommendations, provide assistance, and communicate with other nations regarding the health threat.

PHEIC was declared by the WHO Director for the Influenza Pandemic of 2009–2010 as well as the Ebola epidemic of 2014–2015 and the Zika epidemic in February 2016.

TABLE 3-4 summarizes and compares the IHR as they existed from 1951 until 2007, when the IHR (2005) were implemented.

TABLE 3-4 International Health Regulations Changes		
	1951–2007	**2007-Present**
Scope	Cholera, plague, yellow fever, smallpox (removed after eradication)	Required reporting of PHEIC: not limited to infectious disease
		Detection and containment at source
	Control at borders/ports	
WHO authority	WHO could not initiate an inquiry	WHO can initiate an inquiry based on "unofficial sources" and can ask for additional information from "official sources." WHO can declare a "public health emergency of international concern"
Expectations of member states/nations	Defined capabilities at ports	Set of minimum "core capacities" for detection, reporting, and assessment, with self-reporting of capacity
Consequence of noncompliance with reporting requirements and implementation of "core capacities"	No formal consequences or required external assessment of capacity	No formal consequences or required external assessment of capacity.

(continues)

TABLE 3-4 International Health Regulations Changes		*(continued)*
	1951–2007	**2007-Present**
Coordination of response	No mechanism for coordination of response	WHO expected to provide assistance in response, communicate with other nations, and recommend control measures
International response capabilities	Set of predetermined controls limited to borders and ports	Flexible "evidence-based" responses adapted to the nature of the threat

The IHR are a work in progress. The Ebola epidemic of 2014–2016 highlighted the importance of continuing to improve the IHR. In the 21st century, the international community has begun to respond to the threat of pandemic disease by strengthening the role of the WHO and other international organizations as well as attempting to ensure local capacities. This process will require continuing modifications and enhancements if the world expects to effectively control emerging infections and prevent pandemic diseases.

Health-In-All-Policies That Frames Health as a Single System

A second population health approach to health policy is called **health-in-all-policies**. Health-in-all-polices is grounded in systems thinking. Health-in-all-policies encourages policy makers, whether they are legislators, executive branch officials, private employers, or healthcare providers, to take into account the subtle as well as the obvious impacts of their policies on health.

BOX 3-2 describes an example of health-in-all-policies as it applies to air pollution.

Health policies often require a balance between the rights of individuals and the needs of groups or the society at large. Thus, those who focus on individuals, such as clinicians, may see the world differently from those who focus on population health. This tension between the individual and the society will be seen in the case study of the Elderly Driver.

Health policies for population health represent a broad range of potential interventions. In contrast to the breadth of population health policies, two specific tools of population health require a focused and in-depth understanding. These are screening for disease and risk factor detection, plus vaccination for disease eradication and control. Let's take a look at each of these important tools of population health.

BOX 3-2 Health in All Policies

WHO has developed an example of how health-in-all-policies should work, which is illustrated in **FIGURE 3-4.**[7]

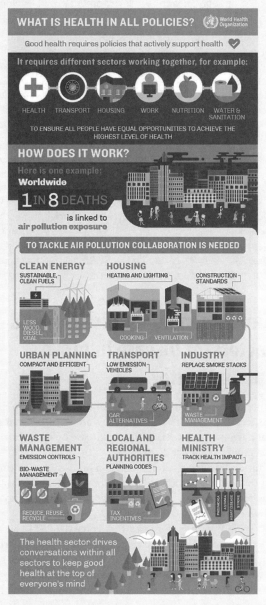

FIGURE 3-4 World Health Organization. What Is Health in All Policies?

Reproduced with permission of the World Health Organization. What is Health in All Policies? Available at: http://who.int/social_determinants/publications /health-policies-manual/HiAP_Infographic.pdf?ua=1. Accessed July 19, 2017.

(continues)

BOX 3-2   Health in All Policies   *(continued)*

In order for health-in-all-policies to be effective, policies adopted by different sectors must reinforce one another. For instance, a health-in-all-policies approach targeting health and development in early childhood may include the following factors:

- Education policies that provide opportunities for women of childbearing age among all income levels to attain a college education or job training
- Substance use and mental health policies that allow children's families to get the support they need
- Employment policies that allow parents to take maternity/paternity leave while maintaining their salary and full health benefits
- Housing policies that require landlords to maintain safe structures free of hazards for young children in order to avoid lead poisoning and asthma triggers

Health-in-all-policies is an overarching framework for integrating health issues into a broad range of social and economic issues. You are likely to hear more about health-in-all-policies as law and policy makers come to better understand the complex relationships between health and social and economic policy.

Many policy makers think about the health-in-all-policies approach through the lens of social determinants of health. Health-in-all-policies requires a careful balancing of fairness between groups and individual versus community rights. Health-in-all-policies confronts decision-makers with difficult questions about fairness and equity that have not often been asked when addressing health issues.

▶ How Can Screening for Diseases and Risk Factors for Disease Improve Population Health?

Screening for disease implies the use of tests on individuals who do not have the symptoms of a specific disease. These individuals are **asymptomatic**. This implies that they do not have symptoms related to the disease being investigated; however, they may have symptoms of other diseases.

Screening for disease can result in detection of disease at an early stage under the assumption that early detection will allow for treatment that will improve outcome. Screening for disease and risk factors have become a common part of population health often integrated into primary care.

The United States Preventive Services Task Force (USPSTF) has developed and applied an evidence-based approach to screening for disease as part of population health often integrated into primary care.[8] The CDC has developed a parallel Community Guide, which includes community- or population-based screening.[9]

These are among the types of recommendations for screening for disease and for risk factors:

- Communicable disease, e.g., hepatitis B and C, HIV
- Cancers, e.g., breast cancer, colon cancer, and melanoma
- Risk factors for cardiovascular disease, e.g., LDL cholesterol, blood pressure, blood sugar

- Disease of pregnancy and the newborn, including a long list of inborn errors of metabolism
- Conditions of childhood development, e.g., hearing, speech and language delay, and vision screening
- Early detection of chronic noncommunicable diseases, e.g., glaucoma and hearing loss
- Early detection of mental health or high-risk behaviors, e.g., alcohol use, opioid use, and high-risk sexual behavior
- Evidence of cognitive changes, e.g., depression and Alzheimer's

Screening for disease and risk factors has become a major way in which population health efforts have been integrated into health care both at the primary care and at specialty levels. Today, these types of screening for disease and risk factors for disease, when based on substantial evidence, have been given a special status in comprehensive health insurance under the ACA. They must be provided without copayment. In other words, individuals do not need to pay a portion of the charges for screening.[†]

It is tempting to try to prevent as many diseases as possible by detecting and addressing risk factors for disease and detecting disease early at a stage when treatment can be most successful. Unfortunately, unless there is strong evidence that screening will be successful, it can do more harm than good by producing false-positive results, submitting patients to costly or dangerous follow-up testing, or by providing false reassurance when false-negative results occur.

Let's take a look at an ideal framework for a successful screening program as well as identify reasons why screening for disease is not universally successful.

Four criteria need to be fulfilled for an ideal screening program.[10] While few, if any, testing and screening programs completely fulfill all four requirements, these criteria provide a standard against which to judge the potential of a screening program. These criteria are as follows:

1. The disease produces substantial death and/or disability.
2. Early detection is possible and improves outcome.
3. There is a feasible testing strategy for screening.
4. Screening is acceptable in terms of harms, costs, and patient acceptance.

The first criterion is perhaps the easiest to evaluate. Conditions such as breast and colon cancer result in substantial death and disability rates. Breast cancer is the second most common cancer in terms of causes of death and is the most common cancer-related cause of death among women in their 50s. Colon cancer is among the most common causes of cancer death in both men and women. Childhood conditions, such as hearing loss and visual impairment, are not always obvious; however, they cause considerable preventable disability.

Determining whether early detection is possible and will improve outcomes is not as easy as it may seem. Screening may result in early detection, but if effective treatment is not available, it may merely alert the clinician and the patient

---

† Under the ACA, screening and other preventive procedures that are recommended—for instance, by a grade of A or B by the USPSTF—do not require that individuals satisfy a deductible or pay a dollar or percentage copayment. This is applicable to all comprehensive insurance as defined by the ACA.

to the disease at an earlier point in time without offering hope of an improved outcome.

Screening cigarette smokers for lung cancer using standard chest X-rays would seem reasonable because lung cancer is the number one cancer killer of both men and women. However, X-ray screening of smokers has not been beneficial in improving the outcome. By the time lung cancer can be seen via chest X-ray, it is already too late to cure. This early detection without improved outcome is called **lead-time bias**.[‡,§]

The third criteria for a successful screening program, a feasible screening strategy, usually requires more than one test. This is the situation since most screening takes place in populations in which the prevalence of the disease or **pretest probability of disease** is 1% or less. When the disease is 1% or less, most positive test results will be falsely positive. That is, they will not correctly indicate the presence of disease.[¶]

For instance, exercise stress tests have been very useful for diagnosis in individuals with symptoms of disease. When used as a screening test on an asymptomatic population with a prevalence of coronary artery disease of 1%, most of the positive test results are false positive. Screening for breast cancer with mammography also produces far more false-positive results than **true-positive** results.

The usual screening strategy is to provide a second test for those with a positive screening test. For mammography, this might be a biopsy. Coronary artery disease might require invasive testing. This approach is called **sequential testing**, or consecutive testing. A sequential testing strategy can usually stop after the first test since

---

‡ The concept of lead time implies that screening produces an earlier diagnosis that may be effectively used to intervene prior to diagnosis without screening. If there is little that can be done to improve outcomes, the extra lead time may result in lead-time bias. It should be noted that a newer screening test for lung cancer, called spiral CT, does meet most of these criteria. Unfortunately, it is very expensive and has only a small impact on the outcome of lung cancer. Therefore, use of spiral CT has become a controversial issue.

§ It is important to distinguish **length bias** from lead-time bias. Like lead-time bias, length bias may create the false impression that early detection improves outcome. Length bias occurs when there are two or more types of a disease with differing rates of progression. When conducting initial screening for early disease, the more slowly progressing type of the disease will be detected more frequently since it remains in the asymptomatic state for a longer period. Disproportionately detecting slowly progressive disease may reduce the impact of early detection since slowly progressive disease often also has much better long-term prognosis, thus reducing the benefit from early detection.

¶ If the test is perfect, i.e., 100% sensitivity and 100% specificity, the pretest probability is not important. The lower the sensitivity and the specificity, the more important the pretest probability of disease. The number of false positives also depends on the cutoff line used to define a positive and a negative test. For many tests, such as blood pressure and LDL cholesterol with a large number of possible test values, a range of normal is used to set these cutoff lines. A range of normal includes the central 95% of the values observed on the test for a population believed to be free of the disease. Thus, the range of normal reflects the way things are, not necessarily the desirable levels on the test. For tests such as blood pressure and LDL cholesterol, where desirable levels are known from long-term follow-up, the desirable range may be substituted in defining a positive and negative test result.

most individuals are negative on the screening test. The second test is only needed for those with a positive screening test.

However, sequential testing misses those who have false-negative results because when a negative test occurs, the testing process is over, at least for the immediate future. Thus, a testing strategy needs to consider how to detect those missed by screening. We need to ask: is there a need for repeat screening, and if so, when should it occur?**

An alternative screening approach, often called **simultaneous testing**, has been used when two types or locations of a disease require two different tests for detection. For many years, this approach was used for colon cancer with sigmoidoscopy used to detect cancer in the sigmoid colon and another test, such as fecal occult blood, being used to detect colon cancer in other locations within the colon. Simultaneous testing may be able to more completely detect a disease if the two tests truly detect different forms of the disease. However, the need for two tests makes for greater effort and greater expense.

Our last criterion for an ideal screening program requires that the screening test be acceptable in terms of harms, costs, and patient acceptance. Harms must be judged by looking at the entire testing strategy, not just the initial test. Physical examination, blood tests, and urine tests are often used as initial screening tests. These tests are virtually harmless. The real question is: what needs to be done if the initial test is positive? If invasive tests, such as catheterization or surgery, are required, the overall testing strategy may present substantial potential harms.

Screenings and diagnostic tests themselves can be quite costly for patients but also for health systems and insurers. Costs are strongly related to the length of time between testing. Testing every year will be far more costly than testing every 5 or 10 years, everything else being equal. The frequency of testing depends on the speed at which the disease develops and progresses, as well as the number of people who can be expected to be missed on the initial test. Mammographic screening needs to be repeated regularly because breast cancer can develop and spread rapidly. In the case of colon cancer, however, longer periods between testing are acceptable because the disease is much slower to develop. Thus, cost considerations may be taken into account when choosing between technologies and when setting the interval between screenings.††

Finally, patient acceptance is key to successful screening. Many screening strategies present little problem with patient acceptance. However, colon cancer screening has had its challenges with patience acceptance because many consider sigmoidoscopy and colonoscopy to be invasive and uncomfortable procedures. Fewer than half the people who qualify for screening based upon current recommendations currently pursue and receive colon cancer screening. This contrasts dramatically

---

** A sequential testing strategy also requires a decision on the order of administering the tests. Issues of cost and safety are often the overriding considerations in determining which test to use first and which to use to confirm an initial positive test.

†† Today, there is a wide range of methods for screening for colon cancer, including occult blood in the stool, colonoscopy, which examines the entire colon, and virtual colonoscopy, which does not require an internal examination. Some newer tests, including DNA testing of stool, are quite accurate but much more costly than testing for occult blood in the stool. Which is the most accurate and cost-effective testing strategy remains controversial. However, the need for and benefits of screening for colon cancer are widely accepted.

with mammography, where a substantial majority of women over 50 now receive the recommended screening.

Screening for disease and for risk factors for disease has been widely accepted in the United States and is usually covered by health insurance when recommended by evidence-based recommendations. Screening can be seen as a success story for the integration of population health efforts into the delivery of health care. However, it is important to recognize the limitations of screening as well as the important role that it plays.

Our final population health tool of the trade is vaccination to prevent disease. Vaccination is used not only to prevent diseases traditionally classified as infectious disease, but also for diseases such as cervical cancer and hepatoma, which have not previously been thought of as infectious diseases. Let's take a look at the important role that vaccination plays in population health.

▶ How Can We Use Population-Based Vaccination for Disease Eradication and Control?

Vaccinations have been a mainstay of population health since Edward Jenner, an English physician, first introduced the practice of inoculation with live cowpox to prevent the development of smallpox at the end of the 18th century. Great progress has been made in developing and using vaccinations since Jenner's day, and hope is often expressed for **eradication** of a wide range of diseases. So far, the only human disease that has been eradicated is smallpox. The eradication of smallpox in the 1970s was a great success and led to the hope that other diseases, especially viruses, could be eradicated as well.

An international campaign has sought to eradicate polio and for years has been on the verge of success but has still not crossed the goal line. Measles, a candidate for eradication that still causes a large number of deaths in developing countries, has been waiting on the sidelines until polio is eradicated.

While eradication remains an important goal of population health, it has been difficult to achieve. At times, unrealistic expectations have been raised for eradication of malaria, TB, and HIV. Let's take a look at the characteristics of a communicable disease that makes it a candidate for eradication. We will also examine how smallpox met nearly all of these criteria, making it an ideal candidate for eradication.

Ideal criteria for eradication and why smallpox met these criteria[11]:

- *No animal reservoir*: Smallpox was an exclusively human disease. That is, there is no reservoir of the disease in animals. It does not affect other species that can then infect additional humans. This also means that if the disease is eliminated from humans, it has nowhere to hide and later reappear in human populations.
- *Short persistence in environment*: The smallpox virus requires human contact and cannot persist for more than a brief time in the environment without a human host. Thus, droplets from sneezing or coughing need to find an immediate victim and are not easily transmitted except by human-to-human contact.

- *Absence of a long-term carrier state*: Once an individual recovers from smallpox, he or she no longer carries the virus and cannot transmit it to others. Smallpox contrasts with diseases such as HIV/AIDS and hepatitis B, which can maintain long-term carrier states and be infectious to others for years or decades.
- *The disease produces long-term immunity*: Once an individual recovers from smallpox, effective immunity is established, preventing a second infection.
- *Vaccination also establishes long-term immunity*: As with the disease itself, the live smallpox vaccine produces very successful long-term immunity. Smallpox did not mutate to become more infectious despite the extensive use of vaccination.
- *Herd immunity protects those who are susceptible*: Long-term immunity from smallpox or from the vaccine made it possible to protect large populations. The aim was at least 80% of the population being vaccinated to interrupt the spread of the infection to the remaining susceptible people.
- *Easily identified disease*: The classic presentation of smallpox is relatively easy to identify by clinicians with experience observing the disease as well as by the average person. This made it possible to quickly diagnose the disease and protect others from being exposed.
- *Effective post-exposure vaccination*: The smallpox vaccine is effective even after exposure to smallpox. This enables effective use of what is called **ring vaccination**.[‡‡]

The presence of all these characteristics makes a disease ideal for eradication. While fulfilling all of them may not be necessary for eradication, the absence of a large number of them makes efforts at eradication less likely to succeed. **TABLE 3-5** outlines these characteristics of smallpox and compares them to polio, the current viral candidate for eradication. It also compares HIV, suggesting that eradication of HIV is most unlikely given our current tools and understandings.

Thus, eradication is often an out-of-reach goal. Nonetheless, vaccination plays an essential role in our population health strategies to control disease from cervical cancer to hepatoma, from meningococcal to pneumococcal disease, and from childhood infections to shingles. Let's see how vaccines can be used to control disease.

▶ How Can Vaccines Be Used to Control Disease Even When Eradication Is Not Feasible?

Vaccines, like any other interventions, need to be assessed to determine their benefits and harms. The benefits as well as the harms of attenuated live vaccines and

---

[‡‡] Ring vaccination for smallpox involves identification of a case of smallpox, vaccination of the individual's household and close contacts, followed by vaccination of all those within a mile radius of the smallpox case. Households within 10 miles were typically searched for additional cases of smallpox. These surveillance and containment efforts were successful even in areas without high levels of vaccination.

TABLE 3-5 Eradication of Human Diseases: Is It Feasible or Should We Focus on Control?

	Smallpox	Polio	HIV/AIDS
Disease is limited to humans (i.e., no animal reservoir)	Yes	Yes	No-animal reservoirs exist
Absence of long-term carrier state	Yes-absent	Yes-absent but may occur in immune compromised	No-carrier state is routine
Vaccination confers long-term immunity And/or effective postexposure	Yes	Yes-but may not be sustained in immune compromised Virus used for live vaccine can produce polio-like illness and has the potential to revert back to "wild type infection"	No-none currently available and will be difficult to achieve
Herd immunity prevents perpetuation of an epidemic?	Yes	Yes	No-large number of previously infected individuals increases the risk to the uninfected

inactivated or killed vaccines, the two currently approved types of vaccines, are quite different. These differences can be outlined as follows[§§]:

Most vaccines are either **attenuated live vaccines** or **inactivated killed vaccines.**[¶¶]

[§§] Vaccination is one type of the broader category known as **immunization**. Immunization includes the administration of preformed antibodies, known as **passive immunity**. Passive immunity today has only limited use, such as protection of pregnant women against specific diseases. Immunization also includes administration of attenuated toxins, such as those produced by tetanus and diphtheria. Antibodies are then produced against the toxin rather than against a virus or bacteria. Vaccines are not limited to protection against viruses and bacteria. A vaccine against malaria, for instance, has shown encouraging results.

[¶¶] A new form of vaccination, known as DNA vaccines, has the potential for effective and inexpensive protection against a wide range of disease. Concerns about the theoretical risk of producing cancer have prevented DNA vaccines from being approved for human use so far. A DNA vaccine, however, has been approved for use in horses to protect against West Nile virus.

Attenuated live vaccines produce a reaction that closely simulates the body's reaction to a viral or bacterial infection. Intercellular as well as extracellular immunity often develops in immunologically competent individuals. However, live vaccines may be contraindicated in individuals who are immune deficient. Attenuated live vaccines often produce long-term immunity and do not require subsequent administration of additional doses or boosters. Live attenuated vaccines have the potential to cross the placenta so that they may be contraindicated in pregnancy. Local and systematic allergic reactions occur, including rare cases of Guillain–Barre Syndrome and anaphylaxis.***

Inactivated killed vaccines are not capable of reproducing and do not produce a reaction that fully simulates the body's reaction to a viral or bacterial infection. The body's reaction is limited to production of antibodies. Inactivated vaccines are safe for those who are immunosuppressed as well as for pregnant women. Unfortunately, inactivated vaccines often do not produce effective immunity, especially in the very young, the very old, and those who are immunosuppressed. Even when vaccination is effective, a booster may be needed. As with attenuated vaccines, local and systematic allergic reactions occur, including rare cases of Guillain–Barre Syndrome and anaphylaxis, which are well documented.

Despite the widespread fears generated by reports of a relationship between vaccinations and autism, the research was found to be fraudulent. There are potential harms from vaccination, but autism is not one of them.

It can be useful when evaluating a vaccine to have a set of ideal criteria, even if these are rare if even realized. A set of ideal criteria for a vaccine is described in **TABLE 3-6**.[12]

Vaccines are as fundamental to population health as drugs are to clinical medicine. Vaccines, like prescription (and nonprescription) drugs, are subject to a comprehensive process of approval by the U.S. Food and Drug Administration, which helps ensure their efficacy. Like drugs, vaccines are rarely 100% effective and at times may be far less effective, such as with the seasonal influenza vaccine, which has varied from less than 20% to approximately 80% effective. At times, vaccines, such as influenza A vaccine, can reduce the severity of illness even when they cannot prevent the disease.

The effectiveness of vaccinations in population health is threatened by an increasing number of individuals who choose not to be vaccinated and are permitted to do so under state laws. In addition, the growing number of immunosuppressed individuals in the population may reduce the effectiveness of vaccines. Today, immunosuppressed populations include the growing number of frail elderly over 85, the large number of individuals living with HIV/AIDS, and the rapidly expanding population taking long-term immune suppressing medication for chronic conditions ranging from rheumatoid arthritis to psoriasis.

The system for reporting adverse effects of vaccines differs greatly from the system for drugs. A no-fault system with financial payment for known adverse effects exists for vaccines. The vaccine side effect reporting system encourages reporting

---

*** A rare but serious complication of a previously used rotavirus vaccine was intussusception leading to life-threatening bowel obstruction. This complication was believed to be due to an overactive response to the vaccine. This vaccine was withdrawn from the market and ultimately replaced with a safer vaccine.

TABLE 3-6 Characteristics of an Ideal Vaccine

Characteristic	Meaning
Good immunological response	In a single dose, produces good antibody- and cell-mediated response, including the site of organism's entry, e.g., respiratory, gastrointestinal, genital
Clinical effectiveness	In practice, provides high levels of protection against the disease and reinfections
Long-term effectiveness	Provides long-term protection without the need for a booster
Immediate effectiveness	Provides immediate protection without extended delay prior to development of immunity
Full-spectrum disease protection	Protection provided against multiple strains of the organism. No evidence of emergence of new strains or increase in strains not included in the vaccine
Few severe adverse effects	Minimal immediate severe adverse effects, such as anaphylaxis; no effects during pregnancy
Ease of administration	No need to freeze or refrigerate
Acceptable route of administration	Route and mode of administration is culturally and ethically acceptable
Allows use of other vaccines simultaneously	Allows simultaneous administration of other vaccines without interfering with effectiveness
Costs of the vaccines are affordable	Costs of the vaccine and its administration reduce the overall cost of care for the disease

Modified from Nelson KE, Williams C. *Infectious Disease Epidemiology: Theory and Practice*. 3rd ed. Burlington, MA: Jones & Bartlett Learning; 2013.

of side effects and means that we usually have reasonably accurate data on the side effects of vaccines.

Population health addresses not only the effectiveness and safety of vaccines, but also how they can be funded, administered, and combined to ensure maximum benefit and minimum harm for large populations.[12]

▶ How Can Vaccines Be Efficiently Administered to Large Populations?

In order to achieve the goal of efficient vaccination of large populations, the development of population or herd immunity, a comprehensive and coordinated approach to vaccination, is needed. Rarely will one approach do the trick. Often, several of these are needed for a successful vaccination effort. These options for implementation have their advantages and disadvantages. **TABLE 3-7** provides a list of options for implementation, their advantages and disadvantages, as well as examples of their use.

The use of vaccines to control disease should not be viewed as a cure-all. Like all interventions, vaccines have their benefits and harms as well as advantages and disadvantages.

TABLE 3-7 Options for Vaccine Administration

	Advantages	Disadvantages	Example
Combination vaccines	Reduce need for multiple visits	Simultaneous live vaccines may reduce effectiveness	Measles, mumps, and rubella (MMR) used successfully despite multiple live vaccines Tetanus, diphtheria, pertussis (TDP) used in combination
Immunization registries	Coordinate efforts and facilitate use of reminder systems	Need for privacy protection	Linkage of birth record, immunization record, and reminder system on the Web
Requirements for school attendance, travel, etc.	Effective if enforced	Coercive	Used widely for entry into elementary school and college May be required for entry to a country, e.g., yellow fever
Mass campaigns	May reach those otherwise unreachable and be key to eradication efforts. Are often cost-effective	More difficult to enforce vaccine indications, contraindications, and ensure follow-up of adverse effects	Used extensively and successfully for smallpox and polio campaigns Increasingly being used in the United States for influenza

(continues)

TABLE 3-7 Options for Vaccine Administration			*(continued)*
Use of vaccine that spreads to others	May reach larger population at low cost	With live attenuated virus such as polio, potential side effects may occur among those who did not consent to vaccination	Live polio vaccine may rarely cause paralytic disease in the nonvaccinated
Use of routes that are less invasive than injection	More acceptable to patient and parents	Often require live vaccines with greater side effects	Nasal spray for influenza was approved for 5-49 year olds but showed low effectiveness
Integrate into care, e.g., hospital discharge or ER	Reach high-risk patients	Requires care coordinate	Pneumococcal vaccine on hospital discharge
Subsidize or cover all costs	Ensures those in need can receive	Cost may be high	If CDC advisory group recommends coverage of a vaccine, then provided without change when recommended but patient uninsured

We have now taken a look at the basic strategies of population health and examined five key tools of the trade of population health. The tools of population health continue to expand. These tools of the trade along with a population health perspective and systems-thinking/systems-doing framework represent the three foundational frameworks of population health.

Knowing what needs to be done is essential to success. Getting the job done, however, requires more than knowing it requires doing. The work of population health requires close connections between the three pillars of population health: health care, public health, and public policy. The principles we have outlined set the stage, but the actors need to work together to make the production a success.

There is increasing interest in population health by clinicians and health administrators, which bodes well for the future. In addition, professions previously seen as nonhealth professions have begun to see themselves as part of the health system. Architects, engineers, urban planners, social workers, foreign services professionals, lawyers, economists, and accountants have roles to play in improving the health of the public. Population health provides a big tent with lots of roles to play and lots of work to do.

🔍 CASE STUDIES AND DISCUSSION QUESTIONS

HIV/AIDS: a Population Health History

Discussion Questions

Return to this case study in the introduction and discuss the following:

1. Which of the basic strategies of population health are illustrated in the case of HIV/AIDS? Explain.
2. Which of the five tools of population health are illustrated in the case of HIV/AIDS? Explain.

Changing Behavior: Cigarette Smoking

It was not going to be easy for Steve to stop smoking. He had been at it for 30 years—ever since he took it up on a dare at age 16 and found that it was a good way to socialize. In his 20s, it seemed to make dealing with the work pressure easier, and in those days, you could smoke in your office and did not even need to shut the door, much less deal with those dirty looks he was getting now.

Steve was always confident that he could take cigarettes or leave them. He would quit when he was good and ready, and a few cigarettes could not hurt. But then he talked to some friends who had quit a decade or more ago and said they would go back in a minute if they thought cigarettes were safe. *Maybe for some people, those cravings just never go away*, he worried to himself. However, there was that bout of walking pneumonia, and then the cough that just did not seem to go away. The cough was so bad that he had trouble smoking more than a few cigarettes a day. The physician assistant let him know that these symptoms were early warning signs of things to come; however, Steve was just not ready to stop. So the physician assistant gave him a fact sheet and let Steve know there was help available when he was ready.

It might have been his fears about his 10-year-old son that finally tipped the scales. "Daddy, those cigarettes are bad for you," he said. Or maybe it was when he found cigarette butts in the backyard after his 16-year-old daughter's birthday party. Steve knew enough to believe that a father who smokes has a child who smokes. So this time, he would do it right.

Steve's physician assistant recognized that Steve was finally ready to quit. He let him know in no uncertain terms that it was important to quit totally, completely, and forever. He also informed Steve that he could rely on help—that he was not alone. With the encouragement of his physician assistant, Steve joined a support group, set a quit date, and announced the date to his friends and family. The new medication he was prescribed seemed to relieve the worst cravings and the feeling he called "crawling the walls."

His wife, Dorothy, was supportive. She cleared the cigarette butts and ashtrays out of the house and dealt with the smell by having all the drapes cleaned. She also helped by getting him up after dinner and taking a walk, which kept him from his old habit of having a cigarette with dessert and coffee. It also helped keep him from gaining too much weight, which she confided was her greatest

(continues)

🔍 CASE STUDIES AND DISCUSSION QUESTIONS *(continued)*

fear. Dorothy's quiet encouragement and subtle reinforcement without nagging worked wonders.

Saving 5–10 dollars a day did not hurt. Steve collected those dollars and put them in a special hiding place. On his first year anniversary of quitting, he wrapped up the dollar bills in a box and gave them to Dorothy as a present. The note inside said: "A trip for us for as long as the money lasts." Dorothy was delighted, but feared the worst when Steve began to open up his present to himself. As he unwrapped a box of cigars, he smiled a big smile and said, "I am congratulating myself on quitting smoking."

Discussion Questions

1. How are each of the phases in the stages of change model illustrated in Steve's case?
2. What effective individual and group approaches are illustrated in this case? Explain.
3. Which effective population health approaches are illustrated in this case? Explain.
4. What is the impact of combining individual clinical approaches with population approaches to cigarette cessation?

The Elderly Driver

It was late in the afternoon on a sunny April day. Maybe it was the sun in her eyes, but 82-year-old Janet found herself in her car in a ditch at the side of the road, unsure of how she got there. Once at the hospital, her son and daughter joined her and heard the good news that Janet had escaped with just a broken arm. The police report strongly suggested that she had swerved off the road, but it was not clear why.

This was not Janet's first driving "episode"; in fact, her driving had been a constant worry to her daughter for over 2 years. Her daughter often offered to take her mom shopping and insisted that she do the driving when they were together. "Don't you trust me?" was the only thanks the daughter received. When alone, Janet continued to drive herself, staying off the freeway and increasingly driving only during the day. She knew it was not as easy as it used to be, but it was her lifeline to independence.

Then, a few months after the April incident, the form for Janet's license renewal arrived. A vision test and a physical exam were required, along with a healthcare professional's certification that Janet was in good health and capable of driving; however, no road test was required. So Janet made a doctor's appointment, and at the end of it, she left the forms with a note for the doctor saying, "To the best doctor I have ever had. Thanks for filling this out. You know how much driving means to me."

On Janet's way home from the doctor's office, it happened. She was driving down the road when suddenly she was crossing that yellow line and heading toward an oncoming car. The teenage driver might have been going a little fast, but Janet was in the wrong lane and the head-on collision killed the 16-year-old passenger in the front seat who was not wearing a seat belt. The 18-year-old driver walked away from the collision unharmed, thanks to a seat belt and an inflated airbag.

Janet was never the same emotionally. And despite escaping the collision with just a few bruises, the loss of her driver's license symbolized the end for her. Those lost weekly shopping trips and the strangers in the assisted living center were not the same as living in her own home. The young man in the collision screaming for help woke her up almost every night. It was only a year after the collision when Janet died, and it was just like she had said: "Take my license away and it will kill me."

Discussion Questions

1. How does this case reflect the important issue of balancing the legal rights of the individual and the rights of society as a whole? Explain.
2. What role do you believe healthcare providers should play in implementing driving laws and regulations? Explain.
3. Identify any changes you would make to prevent the types of outcomes that occurred in this case study. Explain.
4. What aspects from this case study can be applied when addressing the issue of inexperienced young drivers? Explain.

Testing and Screening

Ken had just turned 40, and with a little encouragement from his wife, he decided that it was time to have a physical—it would be his first real visit to a doctor since he broke his arm as a kid. Seeing a doctor had not made sense to him before. He was in great shape, felt fine, and did not smoke.

Maybe it was his 65-year-old father's sudden death from a heart attack just a few weeks after his retirement that finally convinced Ken to find himself a doctor. He knew that his father had had high cholesterol, but he was told his own cholesterol level and electrocardiogram results were okay when he entered the military at age 18. Besides, Ken was not big on desserts and only ate a Big Mac when he took the kids out after their soccer games.

The examination was quite uneventful and Ken was reassured when the doctor could not find anything of concern. A few recommendations on nutrition and better ways to exercise were about all that came out of the visit. Then he got the call from the doctor's office—could he make a follow-up appointment to discuss his cholesterol? His low-density lipoprotein (LDL, or "bad" cholesterol) was 165 and his high-density lipoprotein (HDL, or "good" cholesterol) was 40.

"We used to think these levels were okay because they are so common," his doctor began. "However, now we consider your LDL cholesterol too high because it increases your chances of developing heart and other blood vessel diseases. There is no evidence of heart disease at this point, but your cholesterol needs attention."

"What do you mean by 'attention'?" Ken replied. "I exercise, do not smoke, and generally keep my fats down."

Ken soon learned a lot more about cholesterol. He first tried his best at changing his diet—it helped a little, but just did not do the trick.

Ken's doctor told him: "For some people, there is a strong genetic component to high LDL cholesterol levels, and while diet is still important, it just cannot always

(continues)

🔍 *CASE STUDIES AND DISCUSSION QUESTIONS* *(continued)*

reduce LDL cholesterol enough by itself. Exercise helps, especially by increasing the good cholesterol, but it does not do much for the bad cholesterol. Medication may be needed, and there is now evidence that if taken regularly, it reduces the chances of having a heart attack or at least delays its occurrence."

Taking medication every day was not easy for Ken, but he stuck with the plan. His doctor asked him to have his cholesterol levels checked every few months for the first year. Ken was amazed at how well the medicine worked. His LDL fell from 165 to less than 100 on only a modest dose. In addition to routine cholesterol checks, Ken had his blood tested for potential side effects from the medication, such as impacts to his liver, and he was told to report any long-lasting muscle aches and pains. The good news was that he could not tell he was taking the medication—he felt just fine.

Now that the cholesterol levels had dropped, he thought maybe he could go off the medication if he just watched his diet closely. His doctor let him try that for a month, but after the 30 days were up, his LDL level was back up to 160.

"Looks like you are hooked on medication for life," his doctor said with a wry smile, adding, "At least the extra cost is worth the extra benefit."

Ken and his wife were told the high LDL cholesterol level is a genetic condition. Not only did Ken need to take the medication on a permanent basis, but the pediatrician began testing his kids.

The doctors said, "We are beginning to understand the genetics behind this condition and would like to do some genetic testing on the children, including that new baby of yours."

Ken wondered whether the information on his children's cholesterol levels would be part of their medical records for the rest of their lives. "You are not planning to put the results on the Internet, are you?" Ken joked nervously as they drew blood from his newborn son.

Discussion Questions

1. How does this case study distinguish between the range of normal and the desirable range? Explain.
2. To what extent are the first and second ideal criteria for screening for high LDL cholesterol fulfilled? Explain.
3. To what extent are the third and fourth ideal criteria for screening for high LDL cholesterol fulfilled? Explain.
4. What ethical issues need to be considered in screening for conditions such as elevated LDL cholesterol? Explain.

Influenza in Middleburg and Far Beyond

"New strain of influenza A found in Middleburg," read the headlines in Middleburg, a medium-size Midwestern community. The local, national, and even worldwide Twitter accounts went wild with doomsday scenarios, and Facebook pages were filled with stories on how to hide and histories of relatives who died in the 1918 and 1958 influenza pandemics, which killed more people than any other disease of the 20th century.

Within days, doctor's offices, nurse-run clinics, and emergency rooms in Middleburg were filled with patients with coughs who were convinced they had a deadly disease. Pharmacists were bombarded with questions about what they could do to prevent the disease and what they could do if they had the early signs. Fortunately, only a few cases of the new strain appeared near the end of influenza season, and calm soon returned. The new strain did pose a danger for the coming season but not an immediate threat.

It was ironic that the new strain of influenza A should appear just as Middleburg and the United States were completing the most successful efforts yet to prevent, control, and limit the impact of seasonal influenza, which in the past had often taken 25,000–50,000 lives a year during flu season.

Within weeks, an interagency federal task force, including the Centers for Disease Control and Prevention (CDC), Food and Drug Administration, and the National Institute of Health, was at work developing a plan to address this new threat. They began by looking at what could be learned from the progress that had been made in reducing the number of deaths from seasonal influenza in the United States to below 10,000 and what was needed to confront the potential epidemic to come.

The Task Force found that the work of public health professionals, physicians, physician assistants, nurses, and nurse practitioners, along with pharmacists and pharmaceutical professionals as well as health administrators, had all played a role in this success story, and they all needed to be fully engaged to minimize the impact of the new strain. They also found a need for expanded engagement of the broader community.

The Task Force identified specific examples of changes in recent years that most likely contributed to the reduced impacts of influenza, including the following factors:

- There was better public health surveillance for changes in influenza strains, enabling but not ensuring better matches between the antigens included in seasonal influenza vaccines and the dominant circulating viruses.
- New vaccines were developed by pharmaceutical companies with U. S. governmental support. Some vaccine modifications had already been widely adopted, including those that produce higher antibody levels in those 65 years of age and older; an intradermal vaccine requiring fewer antigens; and a four-component influenza vaccine providing greater protection against influenza B.
- Vaccine effectiveness studies have shown that the intranasal influenza vaccine has not been effective in recent years and has been discontinued based on recommendations of the CDC's Advisory Committee on Immunization Practices, which includes public health and medical professionals with formal relationships, including nursing, physician assistants, health administrators, and pharmacists.
- Increased levels of vaccination resulting from widespread vaccine administration in pharmacies, nurse-run clinics, as well as school-based and community-based vaccine administration.
- Selected use of antiviral drugs for prevention and control has helped, especially in nursing homes, prevent and control outbreaks. Use of antiviral drugs early in the course of influenza may have helped shorten the course of the disease and modestly reduce its spread. Selective use of new rapid diagnostic tests

(continues)

🔍 CASE STUDIES AND DISCUSSION
QUESTIONS   *(continued)*

may have helped in implementing this process, though false negatives are
still frequent.

■ Better workplace precautions and school-based education to reduce the local
spread of influenza.

■ Greater insurance coverage for influenza vaccine in a wide-range of types of
health insurance.

The Task Force report concluded that in the next flu season, the United States
may be faced with an epidemic or even a pandemic from the new influenza strain,
but coordinated population health efforts to prevent, control, and minimize the
impact can save thousands of lives and improve population health.

The Task Force recommended that current efforts need to continue and be
expanded even further in the face of the new influenza strain. They recommended
the use of the following additional efforts by the health and broader community:

■ Aggressive use of recently approved vaccine technology, including cell-
based vaccines and recombinant vaccines that may be more effective, can be
produced more rapidly, and in the case of recombinant vaccines does not use
eggs in its production. These new types of vaccines have recently been shown
to be safe and have efficacy in clinical trials.

■ Early efforts to vaccinate high-risk populations, including healthcare
professionals and nursing home residents.

■ Development of community-based planning for hospital "surge capacity" and
triage procedures, including preparation for a large increase in the need for
intensive care.

■ Planning by local governments, businesses, schools, and healthcare
organizations to implement phased-in efforts to reduce spread, such as school
closings, increased telecommuting, and widespread use of tele-medicine.

■ A coordinated governmental and private communications system needs to
be in place to rapidly get accurate information out to the public and address
rumors and false information.

The leadership and citizens of Middleburg took these recommendations to
heart and took action. With an unusual consensus among community leaders, the
citizens of Middleburg were cautiously optimistic that they were ready for what
might come their way next year.

Discussion Questions

1. Identify types of health professionals needed to reduce the impacts of
   influenza and the role(s) they need to play. Explain.
2. Discuss the roles played by nonhealth professionals and organizations in a
   successful effort to control seasonal or epidemic influenza. Explain.
3. Discuss how this case illustrates the population health strategies of reducing
   high risk and also the improving the average risk. Explain.
4. Discuss the types of population health communication needed to minimize
   the impact of influenza. Explain.

References

1. Weinrich NK. What is social marketing? http://www.social-marketing.com/Whatis.html. Accessed June 18, 2018.
2. Wong F, Huhman M, Asbury L, et al. VERB™—a social marketing campaign to increase physical activity among youth. *Prev Chronic Dis.* 2004;3(1):1-7.
3. Loge, PM. Successful strategic communication: an admonition and five steps. www.peterloge .com/uncategorized/successful-strategic-communication-an-admonition-and-five-steps/. Accessed July 5, 2018.
4. Heath C, Heath D. *Made to Stick: Why Some Ideas Survive and Others Die.* New York: Random House; 2007.
5. Katz R, Fischer J. The revised International Health Regulations: a framework for global pandemic response. *Global Health Governance.* 2010;3(2). http://blogs.shu.edu /ghg/2010/04/01/the-revised-international-health-regulations-a-framework-for-global -pandemic-response/. Accessed June 18, 2018.
6. World Health Organization. Alert, response, and capacity building under the International Health Regulations (IHR). http://www.who.int/ihr/about/10things/en/. Accessed June 18, 2018.
7. World Health Organization. What is health in all policies? http://who.int/social_determinants /publications/health-policiesmanual/HiAP_Infographic.pdf?ua=1. Accessed July 19, 2017.
8. Agency for Healthcare Research and Quality, U.S. Preventive Services Task Force Guide to Clinical Preventive Services. 2002; 1 and 2. AHRQ Pub. No. 02-500.
9. Centers for Disease Control and Prevention. The guide to community preventive services. The community guide. http://www.thecommunityguide.org. Accessed June 18, 2018.
10. Riegelman RK. *Studying a Study and Testing a Test: Reading the Evidence-Based Health Research.* Philadelphia, PA: Lippincott, Williams & Wilkins; 2013.
11. Sompayrac I. *How Pathogenic Viruses Work.* Sudbury, MA: Jones & Bartlett Publishers; 2002.
12. Nelson KE, Williams C. *Infectious Disease Epidemiology: Theory and Practice.* 3rd ed. Burlington, MA: Jones & Bartlett Learning; 2013.

Glossary

Altered environment The impact of chemicals, radiation, and biological products that humans introduce into the environment.

Asymptomatic As used here, the absence of symptoms for a specific disease for which screening is being conducted.

Attenuated live vaccines Use of a living organism in a vaccine. Living organisms included in vaccines are expected to be attenuated or altered to greatly reduce the chances that they will themselves produce disease (synonym: live vaccines).

BIG GEMS A mnemonic that summarizes the determinants of disease, including behavior, infection, genetics, geography, environment, medical care, and socioeconomic-cultural status.

Bottlenecks Factors that limit the effectiveness of systems.

Built environment The physical environment constructed by human beings.

Case–control studies A study that begins by identifying individuals with a disease and individuals without a disease. Those with and without the disease are identified without knowledge of an individual's exposure or nonexposure to the factors being investigated (synonym: retrospective study).

Cohort studies An investigation that begins by identifying a group that has a factor under investigation and a similar group that does not have the factor. The outcome in each group is then assessed (synonym: prospective study).

Collaboration As used here, a form of coordination in which there is joint planning and selective sharing of information.

Community Health Needs Assessment Community-based effort to identify key health needs and issues through systematic, comprehensive data collection and analysis.

Community-Oriented Primary Care (COPC) A structured process designed for community health centers to address community health issues as well as individual health issues.

Culture As used here, multiple economic, religious, and habitual influences on the actions of large numbers of people.

Demographic transition Describes the impacts of falling childhood death rates and extended life spans on the size and the age distribution of populations.

Determinants of health Underlying factors that ultimately bring about disease. Has been referred to as the causes of causes.

Disability-Adjusted Life Years (DALYs) A measure of overall disease burden, expressed as the number of years lost due to ill-health, disability, or early death.

Effectiveness An intervention has been shown to increase the positive outcomes or benefits in the population or setting in which it will be used.

Efficacy An intervention has been shown to increase the positive outcomes or benefits in the population on which it is investigated.

Epidemic A term used when a disease has increased in frequency in a defined geographic area far above its usual rate.

Epidemiological transition Changes in the diseases and conditions producing mortality and morbidity as a result of social and economic development.

Eradication Total elimination of a disease from a human population as well as any animals or ecosystems reservoirs.

Essential Heath Benefits The 10 categories of health services that have been defined as required to ensure that health insurance coverage is considered comprehensive under the Patient Protection and Affordable Care Act (ACA).

Essential Public Health Services The 10 services that have come to define the responsibilities of the combined local, state, and federal governmental public health system.

Etiology The cause of a disease or health condition.

False negative Individuals who have a negative result on a screening test but turn out to have the disease.

False positive Individuals who have a positive result on a screening test but turn out not to have the disease.

Feedback loops In systems analysis, the impact of changes in one influence or factor on other influences or factors in a positive or negative direction.

Health A state of complete physical, social, and mental well-being.

Health-adjusted life expectancy (HALE) A population health status measure that combines life expectancy with a measure of the population's overall quality of health.

Health communications The full range of uses of information in health, from data collection to decision-making.

Health impact assessment A tool that can help communities, decision-makers, and practitioners understand the health impacts of policy changes, even those not intended to affect health.

Health-in-all-policies A comprehensive approach where private and public entities, across sectors, work toward common goals to achieve improved health for all and reduce health inequities.

Health-related quality of life (HRQOL) A health status measure that reflects the number of unhealthy days due to physical plus mental impairment. HRQOL provides an overall quality of health measure, but it does not incorporate the impact of death.

Herd immunity Protection of an entire population from a communicable disease by obtaining individual immunity through vaccination or natural infections by a large percentage of the population (synonym: population immunity).

Human microbiome Microbial organisms that normally live in association with human beings, especially in the gastrointestinal tract.

Immunization The strengthening of the immune system to prevent or control disease through exposure to antigens or administration of antibodies.

Improving-the-average risk A public health approach that assumes that everyone is at some degree of risk and health can be improved by reducing the risk for the entire population.

Inactivated killed vaccine Injection of a nonliving organism or antigens from a pathogen designed to develop antibodies to protect an individual from the disease (synonym: killed vaccine).

Infant mortality rate A population health status measure that estimates the rate of death in the first year of life.

Influences As used in systems thinking, factors or determinants that interact with each other to bring about outcomes, such as disease or the results of disease.

Integration of efforts A form of coordination in which there is joint implementation, including designation of a lead organization.

Interference A term used in systems thinking to describe factors that affect the spread of disease in a population, including spread of noncommunicable diseases.

International Health Regulations A set of internationally accepted rules that allow the World Health Organization to declare a "public health emergency of international concern" and take specific actions to address it.

Interventions The full range of strategies designed to protect health and prevent disease, disability, and death.

Lead-time bias The situation in screening for disease in which early detection does not alter outcome but only increases the interval between detection of the disease and occurrence of the outcome, such as death.

Length bias The tendency of a screening test to more frequently detect individuals with a slowly progressive disease compared with individuals with a rapidly progressive disease.

Leverage points Points or locations in a system at which interventions can have substantial impacts (synonym: control points).

Life expectancy A population health status measure that summarizes the impact of death in an entire population, utilizing the probability of death at each age of life in a particular year in a particular population.

Morbidity A public health term to describe the symptoms produced by a disease or other condition. At times, distinguished from disability, which is defined in terms of function.

Mortality A public health term to describe the frequency of deaths produced by a disease or other condition.

Multiplicative interaction A type of interaction between two or more exposures such that the overall risk when two or more exposures are present is best estimated by multiplying the relative risk of each of the exposures.

Narrowing the spread of the risk curve A possible population health strategy that reduces the risk for high-risk groups while at the same time raising the risk for low-risk groups.

Odds ratio A measure of the strength of the relationship that is often a good approximation of the relative risk. This ratio is calculated as the odds of having the risk factor if the disease is present divided by the odds of having the risk factor if the disease is absent.

One Health The collaborative effort of multiple health science professions, together with their related disciplines and institutions to obtain optimal health for people, domestic animals, wildlife, plants, and our environment.

One Health Educational Framework A framework for education in One Health that includes microbiological influences on health and disease, ecosystem health/physical environment influences, and human–animal interaction.

Pandemic An epidemic occurring worldwide, or over a very wide area, crossing international boundaries and affecting a large number of people.

Parallel play An approach to coordination that requires only shared goals.

Passive immunity Short-term protection against a disease provided by administration of antibodies.

Population Traditionally, the number of individuals living in a geographic area. Today, it is used as a term referring to a defined group of people.

Population dynamics The study of the size and age composition of population and the changes that take place over time.

Population health approach As used here, an evidence-based approach to problem-solving that considers a range of possible interventions, including health care, traditional public health, and social interventions

(synonyms: ecological approach, socioecological approach).

Population health science As used here, an emerging discipline that investigates issues related to population health utilizing a wide range of professionals.

Population health status measures Quantitative summary measures of the health of a large population, such as life expectancy, and HALEs.

Population perspective Here, a focus on the health of the public rather than on the health of one individual at a time.

Population pyramid Graphic display of the size and age distribution of a population divided into males and females.

Pretest probability of disease The probability of the disease before the test results are known. An estimate based on prevalence of the disease, the presence of risk factors for the disease, and, if present, signs or symptoms suggestive of the disease.

Primary intervention An intervention that occurs before the onset of the disease.

Public health emergency of international concern A formal statement by the Director of the World Health Organization that may be issued under the International Health Regulations.

R naught (R_0) The number of new cases one individual with the disease generates on average over the course of the disease's communicable period (synonyms: reproduction number, reproduction ratio).

Randomized controlled trial An investigation in which individuals are assigned to study or control groups using a chance process of randomization (synonym: experimental study).

Reducing high risk A population health strategy that focuses on groups with higher than average risk or probability of a negative outcome.

Relative risk A ratio of the probability of the outcome if a factor known as a risk factor is present compared to the probability of the outcome if the factor is not present.

Ring vaccination As used in the smallpox eradication program, immediate vaccination of populations in surrounding geographic areas after identification of a case of disease.

Risk factor A characteristic of individuals or an exposure that increases the probability of developing a disease. It does not imply that a contributory cause has been established.

RNA virus A virus that has ribonucleic acid as its genetic material.

Screening As used here, testing individuals who are asymptomatic for a disease as part of a strategy to diagnose a disease or identify a risk factor.

Secondary intervention Early detection of disease or risk factors and intervention during an asymptomatic phase.

Sequential testing A screening strategy that uses one test followed by one or more additional tests if the first test is positive (synonym: consecutive testing).

Simultaneous testing A screening strategy that uses two tests initially, with follow-up testing if either test is positive (synonym: parallel testing).

Social determinants of health The complex, integrated, and overlapping social structures and economic systems, including the social environment, physical environment, health services, and structural and societal factors.

Social marketing The use of marketing theory, skills, and practice to achieve social change. Use and extension of traditional product marketing to population health.

Stages of change model A model of behavioral change that hypothesizes five steps in the process of behavioral change, including precontemplation, contemplation, preparation, action, and maintenance (synonym: transtheoretical model).

Straight line relationship An association in which the dependent variable increases or decreases by the same amount as the extent of exposure to the independent variable increases

or decreases. As used here, implies that the magnitude of the relative risks can be added together (synonym: linear relationship).

System An interacting group of items forming a unified whole.

System error Problem resulting from deficiencies in the system for delivering health care or other services.

Systems analysis A variety of methods that operationalize the investigation of systems.

Systems doing As used here, indicates three basic types of coordination between components of the health system: parallel play, collaboration, and integration of efforts.

Systems-thinking An approach that examines multiple influences on the development of an outcome or outcomes and attempts to bring them together in a coherent whole.

Tertiary intervention An intervention that occurs after the initial occurrence of symptoms but before irreversible disability occurs.

True positive Individuals who have a positive result on a screening test and turn out to have the disease.

Unaltered environment The natural environment.

Under-5 mortality A population health status measure that estimates the probability of dying during the first 5 years of life.

Vaccination A preparation of killed pathogen or living attenuated pathogen that is administered to produce or artificially increase immunity to a disease. Immunization is often used as a synonym, but it also includes passive protection with antibodies as well as administration of toxins.

Victim blaming Placing the responsibility or blame for a bad outcome on the individual who experiences the bad outcome due to his or her behavior.

Index

Page numbers followed by *f, t* and *b* indicate figures, tables and boxes, respectively.

M

N

O

P